Dr. Tom Linden's Guide to Online Medicine

Tom Linden, M.D.
Michelle L. Kienholz

McGraw-Hill

New York   San Francisco   Washington, D.C.   Auckland   Bogotá
Caracas   Lisbon   London   Madrid   Mexico City   Milan
Montreal   New Delhi   San Juan   Singapore
Sydney   Tokyo   Toronto

pbk   1 2 3 4 5 6 7 8 9 FGR/FGR 9 0 0 9 8 7 6 5

Library of Congress Cataloging-in-Publication Data
Linden, Tom.
   Dr. Tom Linden's guide to online medicine / Tom Linden, M. D. & Michelle
L. Kienholz.
     p   cm.
   Includes index.
   ISBN 0-07-038055-4 (p)
    1. Medicine—Computer network resources. 2. Internet (Computer
network) 3. Database searching. I. Kienholz, Michelle L.
   II. Title.
   R859.7.D36L56   1995
   025.06'61—dc20   95-31555
                                                          CIP

Editorial team: Brad Schepp, Acquisitions Editor
                Kellie Hagan, Book Editor
                Robert E. Ostrander, Executive Editor
Production team: Katherine G. Brown, Director
                Susan E. Hansford, Coding
                Ollie Harmon, Coding
                Toya B. Warner, Computer Artist
                Wanda S. Ditch, Desktop Operator
                Nancy K. Mickley, Proofreading
                Jodi L. Tyler, Indexer
Design team: Jaclyn J. Boone, Designer
             Katherine Lukaszewicz, Associate Designer

BR1*
0380554

To Cindy, for her love and support; to Sarah, for the joy she brings to the world; to my mother and father, for their years of love and caring.

To my mother and my husband, who have loved and supported me through so much.

Contents

Part II: Where to find online medical resources

Part III: How to use online medical information

Acknowledgments

No book represents the efforts of the authors alone. We have several people to thank for their help.

We'd like to thank Bill Adler for getting the ball rolling and developing the concept for this book. Thanks also to McGraw-Hill acquisitions editor Brad Schepp, his assistant Stacey Spurlock, and senior editor Kellie Hagan for shepherding the manuscript through the publishing process. We also appreciate the work of assistant art director Lori Schlosser in developing the cover design.

Thanks to Mark Bisgeier for getting Tom Linden plugged into the Internet, to Wayne Liebman for sharing his love of the English language, and to Cindy Rogers for her consulting, cheerleading, typing, and legal skills. Particular thanks go to Barbara Maines and the Central Rappahannock Regional Library for bringing the Internet to Michelle Kienholz and the rest of Montross, and to Robert Pawlak, Ph.D. for his patience and invaluable technical support.

We're grateful to Janine Dunne (America Online), Debra Young (CompuServe), Gwenn Gauthier (Delphi), Kim Upham (e•World), Pam Angelus (GEnie), and Brian Elk (Prodigy) for helping us explore their services.

Acknowledgments

We must especially thank all the online citizens who took time to share their thoughts and experiences with us. Thanks also to all the people committed to making online health information and support available to the world.

Finally, thanks to all those who allowed us to use illustrations of their online sites, in particular the following:

AIDS Info BBS
Stephen M. Borowitz, M.D., University of Virginia
Kairos Support for Caregivers
Deborah K. Levine, Columbia University
Marlene M. Maheu, Ph.D., Executive Editor, Self-Help Psychology Magazine
Gary Malet, D.O., Medical Matrix, Internet Working Group of the American
    Medical Informatics Association
Mind Gear Inc.
Health Sciences Information Systems Integration, University of Washington
Andrew Patrick, Ph.D., Network Services & Interface Design Laboratory,
    Communications Research Centre, Industry Canada
William L. Robertson
Janne Sinkkonen, Cognitive Psychophysiology Research Unit, University
    of Helsinki
Andy Spooner, M.D.
Atlanta Reproductive Centre, Dr. Mark Perloe
Duke University Student Health Education
Nigel P. Bamford, M.B., alt.support.stop-smoking
John F. Murphy, M.D.
Brian Pinkerton
Prodigy Services Company

Introduction

Many books about online services are outdated by the time they're published, and they try to cover so much ground that they don't cover anything. The language is often intimidating, with arcane details only a computer geek could love.

Dr. Tom Linden's Guide to Online Medicine is different. We've looked at the online world and seen it through a patient's eyes—quite literally. While writing this book, one of us celebrated the birth of a child; the other had an emergency appendectomy. We've both turned to online medical resources for information and advice in our lives and our jobs.

To research the book, we've visited hundreds of online medical sites and met dozens of wonderful Internet citizens along the way. Through this guide, you'll see what we've seen and hear the stories of others who have ventured online for health information and support.

We believe you'll find this information invaluable. Your disease or condition might prevent you from going out, either to the library to do research or to a support group for a morale boost. You might live too far from a city to even have these options. You might feel helpless, not in control of your medical care. Getting online will put you back in control—back in charge of your treatment, your health, and your life.

Dr. Tom Linden's Guide to Online Medicine will help you tap the vast online storehouse of medical and health information. In this book, we'll guide you to the best resources accessible via the Internet, commercial online services, and bulletin board systems (BBSs) around the world, and we'll tell you how to share what you learn with your doctor. With this guide, you'll learn how to find health information simply, quickly, and inexpensively. In short, we'll show you how to:

➤ Perform online searches for specific medical topics

➤ Subscribe to electronic medical newsletters and mailing lists

➤ Track down experts on even the most obscure maladies

➤ Post messages that get results

➤ Find support from other people with the same condition

➤ Get information about new and ongoing clinical trials

➤ Explore both traditional and alternative therapies

➤ Conduct research for academic and popular medical writing

➤ Keep track of late-breaking medical news

➤ Locate specialized health information for children, older adults, women, men, and minorities

➤ Find sources of information in all fields of medicine

Part one of *Dr. Tom Linden's Guide* explains how to access the Internet and major online services. If you have a computer and modem but haven't decided which commercial service to join, we'll help you survey the medical and health offerings for each. If the Internet intimidates you, rest easy. We'll show you how to tackle it, introducing you to the tools that will help you find medical information.

Introduction

Tired of monthly online subscription fees? Try a BBS, which will be kinder to your wallet. Many BBSs are free, or require only modest annual subscription fees. Some even have toll-free access numbers. Most offer medical resources, including databases and message boards. We'll tell you which medical BBSs are the best and where to find them.

So now you're online. Where do you go for the medical information you need? In part two, *Where to find online medical resources*, we take you through the maze of health resources. We tell you where to find information about AIDS (chapter 6), cancer (chapter 7), neurologic disorders (chapter 9), disabilities (chapter 14), and many other diseases and medical conditions (chapter 8).

We devote an entire chapter to mental health and psychology (chapter 10), with specific directions on where to find online information about addiction, alcoholism, attention deficit disorder, depression, drug abuse, grief, mood disorders, schizophrenia, sexual abuse, smoking cessation, and suicide. We describe online psychological and psychiatric services as well as discussion and support groups.

Suppose you have a root canal that fails. Worried about what kind of filling to get? How to find a good dentist? In chapter 11, *From teeth to toes*, we review the leading dentistry sites where you can find the latest on dental, periodontal, and preventive dentistry care.

What if you spend too much time at the computer and develop a repetitive strain injury such as carpal tunnel syndrome? In the section in chapter 11 on occupational medicine, you'll find where to get information to keep the situation from getting worse. The answers to your problems might reside on one of several World Wide Web (WWW) pages or any of a number of mailing lists, which are e-mail discussion groups on the Internet.

If you think you are what you eat, then take a look at the nutrition section, also in chapter 11, where you'll find sites on everything from fat-free foods to a veggie mailing list.

Introduction

In part three, *How to use online medical information*, we offer strategies for getting the most from your healthcare information quest. We give pointers on how to critically evaluate what you find online, warn of hazards along the way, and give advice on how to approach your doctor with the information you find. Although this guide won't replace your personal physician, it will enable you to become a more informed medical consumer.

Finally, to help healthcare professionals reach their colleagues directly and easily, we offer an appendix of online resources not meant for casual use. Because researchers have long used the Internet to exchange information, there are more resources for academic and clinical health professionals than for patients and the general public.

That's a quick look at *Dr. Tom Linden's Guide to Online Medicine*. In the pages that follow, we hope to guide you toward where you need or want to go. Sit back, get comfortable, and enjoy the ride!

1
The Internet

*T*o get started on the Internet, you don't need to be a computer expert or even understand how the Internet works. As with many computer-related skills, you'll learn most quickly by signing on and experimenting. After you've spent time online, you might want to visit your public library or purchase a comprehensive Internet reference to help you explore further (we suggest a few in appendix A). You'll also find plenty of help online; most bulletin board systems (BBSs) and commercial services offering access to the Internet also maintain message boards, libraries, live discussions, and other means of communicating about and explaining cyberspace.

Electronic mail

Electronic mail (e-mail) is the most common connection people have with the Internet. You can send messages all over the world with a dedicated electronic mailbox, a BBS account, a commercial online service subscription, a network terminal (at a business or university), or an Internet service provider. How you send and receive e-mail depends on the type of account you have. If you have a question about how to address e-mail to a specific location, most general Internet books can provide answers.

You might find lowly e-mail to be your best online medical resource. Even if it's your only link to the Internet, you'll still be well connected. You can subscribe to mailing lists, write to health organizations for information, and communicate with medical experts. Using e-mail alone, you can use other Internet features, including file transfer protocol (FTP), World Wide Web (WWW), and gopher.

Why look to the Internet for medical information?

Whether you're searching for health information or support, you have access to a greater selection of resources than you'll find in one institution alone. There are opportunities to ask people with varied experiences and backgrounds for "second opinions" on health problems. The online community is altruistic. Rarely will a plea for information or advice go unanswered. There's no intimidation, no face-to-face confrontation, but beware the dangers of unofficial advice.

- What can you expect to find? As the medical profession latches on to the Internet, you can expect to find the same information your doctor has. That is, of course, if you aren't talking online to him or her first.

- Finding it difficult to keep up? Don't go to a university library. Subscribe to the Journal Watch mailing list.

- Need to give a case presentation on a particular kind of cancer? Visit one of my favorite resources, the CancerNet database.

- Suffering from or studying HIV? Read what's topical in Usenet's sci.med.aids.

- Want to teach your children CPR? Use FTP to get free tutorial software from one of many medical software repositories.

- Don't know where to find information on anesthetics? Go to gopher://gasnet.med.nyu.edu:70/1.

- What about the Web? Visit the Virtual Hospital.

These are only some of many resources that can put information you need in your hand. No doubt you'll discover many more as you browse the pages of Dr. Tom's guide.

How do you become involved?

If you're starting out with computers and modems, you might already have discovered that telecommunicating is a bit trickier than using a word processor. That's why I recommend learning about online services by joining a local bulletin board (BBS) with an easy-to-use graphical interface. The skills you learn there will be invaluable when you tackle the Internet. Many smaller BBSs and larger commercial services offer some form of Internet connectivity, such as e-mail, mailing lists, and the Usenet. This allows you to learn about the Internet in a familiar and friendly environment and find out what others are doing by reading newsgroups. Jumping head-first into the Internet is a recipe for confusion and disinterest. Remember that online services aren't all alike. Find one that fits you.

Where's the interesting stuff?

Some people are no doubt put off by descriptions of the Internet as a data dump. It's mind-boggling big, but there is quality, not just quantity. It can be unproductive to simply browse using Gopher or the Web. What you need is a focused guide (like this book) that helps direct you toward what you're looking for. Another good place to start is a document pointing to other resources, such as a FAQ (frequently asked questions) file. Aside from containing pointers, many FAQs are written by enthusiastic people answering the questions most relevant to patients. There are also a number of excellent home pages on the Web that do the same, such as Medical Matrix.

Dr. Bruce C. McKenzie
bruce-m@cybertas.demon.co.uk

Usenet newsgroups

Usenet (short for *user's network*) is a large network of newsgroups, which are similar to message centers or bulletin boards. In newsgroups, people congregate online to converse about hundreds of topics related to a central theme.

Some newsgroups are moderated, meaning every posted message is approved by one or more moderators, usually experts in their fields. Moderated newsgroups are generally better organized and more civil than unmoderated groups. As with e-mail, how you subscribe, read, and reply to a newsgroup depends on your type of access—whether it's a BBS echo, a commercial service, or an Internet service provider.

The sci groups, such as sci.med or sci.psychology, offer forums for information exchange and scientific discussion, including the debate over healthcare issues. The misc.health groups are similar but have a more patient-oriented tone. For sharing and caring, go to the alt.support groups, such as alt.support.cancer or alt.support.allergy. Sometimes more than one group covers the same disorder, with each group offering a different perspective (e.g., alt.support.arthritis and misc.health.arthritis). Finally, some newsgroups share messages from mailing lists, such as bit.listserv.deaf-l. This allows you to interact with mailing list members without subscribing.

In part two, *Where to find online medical resources*, we'll list relevant medical newsgroups for specific diseases and disorders. To find a group that deals with a topic that interests you, type a keyword in your newsreader program. If you're unfamiliar with newsgroups and want more information about how they work, check news.announce.newusers.

One of the best features of a newsgroup is its FAQ (frequently asked questions) file. Posted on a regular basis, a FAQ answers basic questions, suggests online and offline resources for more information, outlines rules adopted by the newsgroup, and reminds members about their online responsibilities. The FAQ author usually identifies his or her qualifications, sometimes appending a bibliography. FAQs might also be available through related Web sites.

Mailing lists

If you like receiving mail, you're in luck. Subscribe to a couple of mailing lists, and your e-mailbox will never be empty. However, even a few mailing list subscriptions can unleash a flood of e-mail. That can lead to added costs if your

```
┌──────────────────────────────────────────────────────────────┐
│ ▬       CompuServe Information Manager              ▼ ▲ │
├──────────────────────────────────────────────────────────────┤
│  File   Edit   Help                                            │
│ ─────────────────────────────────────────────────────────     │
│                          Browse                                │
│                  Newsgroup: sci.med                            │
│                                                                │
│     Thread                                        Articles     │
│     ┌──────────────────────────────────────────────────┐ ┌─┐ │
│     │ APLASTIC ANEMIA                               1   │ │▲│ │
│     │ ASA                                           1   │ └─┘ │
│     │ Aspirin, heart attacks, and statistics - INTERNET NEWS FLASH 3 │ │
│     │ Aspirin, heart attacks, etc.                  1   │     │
│     │ Asthma Question                               1   │ ▓   │
│     │ Atten: ID specialists/Cardiologists           1   │ ▓   │
│     │ Australia: can a Yank doctor practice there? Is it practi... 1 │ │
│     │ BCG Vaccine                                   2   │ ┌─┐ │
│     │ Beijing-Help on diagnosis for coma patient please 1 │ │▼│ │
│     └──────────────────────────────────────────────────┘ └─┘ │
│                                                                │
│   ┌────────────────────────┐   ┌──────────┐   ┌──────────┐   │
│   │ ⦿ As is                │   │   Get    │   │  Create  │   │
│   │ ○ Quoted  ┌──────────┐ │   └──────────┘   └──────────┘   │
│   │           │ Retrieve │ │                                  │
│   │           └──────────┘ │   ┌──────────┐   ┌──────────┐   │
│   └────────────────────────┘   │  Clear   │   │  Cancel  │   │
│                                 └──────────┘   └──────────┘   │
│                                                                │
└──────────────────────────────────────────────────────────────┘
```

You can easily scan Usenet newsgroup threads by using a graphical reader such as the one offered by CompuServe.

Internet provider is a toll call away or if it limits the number of free messages you can receive.

Some mailing lists are also available as Usenet newsgroups, often identified by a bit.listserv name. To avoid excessive e-mail, you might want to read the newsgroup instead. On the other hand, if you don't have access to newsgroups, mailing lists offer a great resource. As with newsgroups, mailing lists can be either moderated or unmoderated.

Many list owners use automated computer programs, such as Listserv or Majordomo, to handle routine tasks. When you subscribe, you'll receive infor-

– 5 –

mation on how to participate. Please note the following major automated commands, which you type in the message body, not the subject line:

```
SUB (or) SUBSCRIBE listname yourfirstname yourlastname
UN (or) UNSUBSCRIBE (or) SIGNOFF listname
HELP
INFO ?
```

Sending the SUBSCRIBE or UNSUBSCRIBE commands will put your name on or off a mailing list, respectively. Sending the HELP command will generate a reply telling you whether the mailing list supports a digest option (one big message), an index option (which allows you to select individual messages to read), or other shortcuts to make participation easier. Sending the INFO ? command will generate a list of topics for which information is available. You might also be able to send the command INFO FAQ to retrieve the list's FAQ.

Not all mailing lists are automated. To join a list, sometimes you'll need to send a brief request via e-mail to the person who owns and operates the list. Read the description of the list before joining to save the time and bother of having to unsubscribe if the list doesn't meet your needs. Once you subscribe, be sure to save the information describing how to unsubscribe if you decide the list no longer meets your needs.

File transfer protocol (FTP)

The file transfer protocol allows you to download software, text, audio, and graphic files from computers all over the world. Newsgroups and mailing lists often maintain FTP sites for their archives, important documents (like FAQs), and other files. Much medical information is available through anonymous FTP, which means you don't need a user name and password to gain access to the computer on which the files are stored.

Retrieving files can be as easy as copying them into a PC or Macintosh, or as cumbersome as using UNIX commands. Don't be afraid to practice with whatever software you have, but limit your practice time to evenings and weekends, when most FTP sites are least busy. If you plan to use FTP a lot and don't have a point-and-click interface, consult a general Internet book to learn about the types of files and compression software available.

Of course, with millions of FTP files from which to choose, you'll need to know what you want and where to find it. Fortunately, your friend Archie will help you. Archie is a program that searches files based on a keyword, filename, directory name, or group of characters. Different Archie programs require different amounts of information. When using Archie, you need to be as specific as possible, or you might get thousands of potential matches to your search request.

How you get to Archie depends on how you get to the Internet. Some providers include a link to Archie in their directories. You can use telnet to connect to an Archie site (such as archie.sura.net or archie.unl.edu), or you can send e-mail (archie@archie.sura.net or archie@archie.unl.edu). If you send e-mail, type HELP in the subject line to get instructions.

You might need Archie at some point if the FTP site you've been using moves. This happens when an FTP site becomes overburdened by the requests it receives. The files are sometimes rearranged and moved to accommodate the increased activity. If you don't get a message telling you the new FTP address, ask Archie.

While you shouldn't be afraid to use FTP to get files, be wary of ripping into those files as soon as they hit your hard drive. A computer virus can infect executable files (software). Most documents can't be infected, but be sure to check them too. The volunteers at some FTP sites screen submitted files for viruses, but you cannot and should never count on this. If you plan to download medical files from the Internet, install anti-virus software in your computer. Doctor's orders.

Gopher

Gopher servers organize information like folders in a filing cabinet. Inside each labeled folder you'll find individual files—maybe more folders—or maybe tel-

Gopher Menu

- INDEX to Health Services
- Cancer
- Drugs, Alcohol, & Smoking
- Eyes & Skin
- General
- Introduction to the Women's Health Exam
- Nutrition
- Sexual Concerns
- Women's Health Exam

Gopher directories include folders, text files, search tools, and other options, such as telnet connections.

net connections to other online resources. In addition, many medical gophers have links to other gophers around the world. For example, you can go to the National Institute of Allergy and Infectious Diseases' gopher server to look for AIDS information. If you find an interesting folder and click on it, you might find yourself transparently transported to AIDS-related gopher servers in San Francisco (AIDS Info BBS), Amsterdam (HIVNET), or Switzerland (Global Programme on AIDS)—all without having to enter another address.

Sometimes the connections aren't so seamless, especially when you're accessing gophers in Europe, Asia, and Australia. If your gopher software can't connect to a particular gopher server, it will usually give up after a few minutes. The remote computer might be turned off, too busy, or having other problems. Be prepared for delays, especially during U.S. daytime hours.

To make your gopher time more efficient, try using a couple of search programs. Veronica searches gopherspace to locate menu titles that match a keyword you supply. When you arrive at particularly large gopher servers, you'll often have the option Search This Gopher. If you want to find a file that contains a keyword in the text itself, use WAIS (wide area information servers ....), which indexes thousands of online documents around the world, including some documents not accessible by gopher. The search might be as easy as typing a few keywords. On the other hand, you might need to know particular commands and specify which database you'd like WAIS to search. The ease of your search depends on the type of software you have.

World Wide Web (WWW)

As easy as gopher is to use, the World Wide Web is even easier. Take the following example. Suppose you're on a gopher server and reading a document about Type I diabetes. Within the document you see a reference to an insulin pump. To find more about that pump, you need to close the diabetes document to search for another document, another folder, or even another gopher server that contains the information you need.

In contrast, on the Web, the Type I diabetes document might have a link to another document that reviews the pump. Simply clicking on the words *insulin pump* in the original document will transfer you to the second document, which might be in the same folder or on another computer on the other side of the world. With the Web, there's no need to open and close files and folders. Just point and click.

Not every word in every Web document offers these links. Only files written in HTML (hypertext mark-up language) allow you to move from site to site, or document to document. You'll recognize the linked words or phrases because they're formatted differently—either underlined, typed in bold or a different color, or numbered (usually in brackets). This hypertext feature is what sets the Web apart from every other Internet service and makes it so easy to use. Because you jump or browse around the Web, the software you use to access this information is called a *browser*.

In addition to its own vast resources, the WWW also connects to gopher servers, FTP sites, Internet relay chat (IRC), telnet, newsgroups (depending on your browser), and other Internet features. On the Web, you have access to graphics, video, and sound. Every day more interactive medical text books and case studies come online. These teaching tools offer x-rays and other medical images, photos or videos of patients, sounds (such as heart rhythms), and other teaching devices.

If you've just started researching a medical topic, you'll find the Web particularly useful since you can quickly scan the landscape. Beware, however. You might find yourself sucked in, moving around stream-of-consciousness style, before you realize several hours have passed. Take a few practice runs to explore, but also take time to focus your search. If you use a graphical Web browser, navigating the Web can be slow, especially when viewing many images and traveling during peak hours. You can skip around much faster if you search with a text-only browser like Lynx or turn off the graphics option of your Web browser.

If you're on the Web and know where you want to go, the quickest way to get to your destination is to simply type the URL (universal resource locator). The URL is the address that starts with http:// or gopher:// or ftp://. If you don't have an address, you can use one of several catalogs or search engines, which we describe in chapter 15, *Searching for medical resources.* Once you've located a site of interest, you might want to add it to your list of bookmarks. That way you don't have to type its URL each time you want to access it.

Internet relay chat (IRC)

If you use a commercial online service, you're probably familiar with chat or conference rooms where you "talk" in real time with other people who have "entered" the same room. With IRC, you meet in international chat rooms, known as *channels*. Different groups use different channels, named to reflect the channel's users or purpose. Not surprisingly, IRC is especially helpful for people who want support and live interaction with others, such as individuals dealing with depression or recovering from addiction. (For example, if you want to talk to people involved in a 12-step recovery, the channel is #12step.) Channels are usually available day or night. Support groups also schedule regular IRC meetings, often with a moderator and a defined discussion topic. Newsgroups that use this IRC feature regularly post information about schedules, commands, and protocol. Some Web pages and gopher servers also contain documents with this scheduling information.

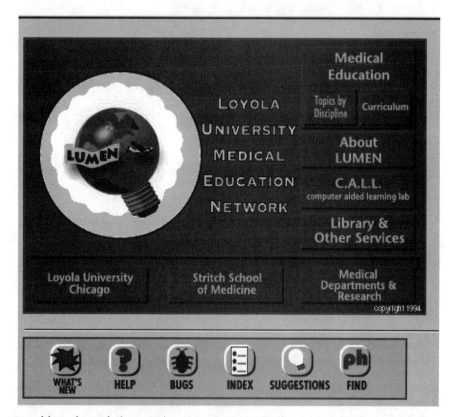

World Wide Web (WWW) pages are most easily accessed with graphical browsers.

Telnet

Telnet allows you to use a remote computer as though it were on your desktop. To sign on, you need a user name and password. If you use a telnet connection available through a gopher server or Web page, you'll usually get instructions for logging on. Most medical libraries offer a telnet connection that leads to catalog information but not actual text from books or journals.

2

Local online services

Bulletin board systems (BBSs)

*I*f the size, scope, or expense of the Internet or even a commercial online service overwhelms you, then you might prefer a local BBS. The site is more intimate, and the tone is often friendlier and more supportive. In areas where you must dial long distance to reach the Internet, you might find a BBS within your telephone exchange. Bulletin board systems differ widely in what they offer. On some BBSs, you can send and receive Internet e-mail and read Usenet newsgroups. In later chapters we review a few of the hundreds of medical BBSs offering medical discussion groups, files, and software.

```
        File areas available:

 1) NIH INFORMATION INDEX        2) NIH PUBLICATIONS
 3) NIH PRESS RELEASES           4) HEALTHLINE & NEWS AND FEATURES
 5) NIH CALENDARS                6) NIH IMAGES
 7) NIH ALMANAC                  8) NIH HISTORY
 9) CLINIC ALERTS               10) UTILITIES
11) FULL TEXT HEALTH PUBLICATIONS 12) NIH JAMA COLUMNS
13) ENVIRONMENTAL CONCERNS      14) OFFICE OF ALTERNATIVE MEDICINE
15) NIH CONSENSUS STATEMENTS    16) NIH TECH ASSESSMENT STATEMENTS

File area [1-16], [L]ist, [H]elp, [Q]uit, [ENTER = All]?
```

National Institutes of Health Information Center

Bulletin board systems (BBSs) offer numbered lists of options.

For a description of a huge network of more than 30,000 BBSs called Fidonet, we turn the discussion over to a dedicated BBS user. If you're already online and read sci.med/Grand_Rounds or many other newsgroups, you might recognize this contributor.

Fidonet BBSs

If you have a personal computer, communications software, and a modem, you can probably access BBSs in your area. For a list of BBSs, look in computer magazines, especially *Boardwatch Magazine*, or free local computer papers. Once you connect with a BBS, you'll learn about others. While some BBSs charge users a nominal fee for full access, most Fidonet BBSs are free.

All BBSs are unique in what they provide. Most offer files and message areas, called *echoes* on Fidonet. Some echoes are local, meaning only users of the BBS holding the discussion can participate. There are also echoes that pertain only to a particular city or local area. Then there are national echoes, which might be picked up by BBS sysops (system operators) anywhere in the world. If you know of a national echo you want to read, ask your sysop. Sysops are usually happy to bring in more echoes.

To help understand echoes better, think of them as telephone party lines where many people are listening. When you send a message, it travels from system to system throughout the world. Messages might take up to a week to reach BBSs in Australia, Germany, or elsewhere; and a reply can take as long. However, new satellite technology is reducing sending and receiving time.

With a simple communications program, you can access a BBS to read messages in any echoes that interest you. Before calling a BBS, set your communications software to the most common settings: 8 data bits, no parity, and 1 stop bit. This allows your modem to communicate with the BBS modem properly. When you first connect, the BBS will ask you to fill out a questionnaire. Once the sysop verifies who you are, you need enter only your name and password when signing on. Most BBSs allow users to spend about one hour per day online.

– 13 –

Most BBSs also have a help area to teach you how to move around the system, and sysops are usually willing to provide assistance. If you really enjoy BBSing, you can download software to call up the BBS and quickly download your mail (including messages from the echoes) before signing off. The software will then sort your messages into folders (by echo) so you can read them at your leisure, write your responses, create new messages, and send them back to the BBS. This method is more complicated and requires a better understanding of the network, but you'll catch on.

BBSing is fun. But, in my humble opinion, each BBS should have an announcement as you sign on that says: "Warning: BBSing is addictive!"

Linda Cummings

Freenets

Freenets bring together the best of two worlds—the sense of community and friendliness of a local BBS with the range of forums of a commercial service. Some freenets also include access to the Internet. Freenets are electronic villages that provide information and support tailored to residents of a particular geographic area. They offer many resources, including community news, library programs, political issues, and weather. Most freenets maintain a health center or medical arts building, constructed like a forum on a commercial service with places to ask health-related questions, share support in small groups, and retrieve information about common medical topics. They also typically announce public health information, such as when a local clinic is open or when offline parenting classes are held.

Many Internet books list modem numbers and telnet addresses (and login terms) for freenets in the United States and Canada. For the latest details on available freenets, dial 216-247-6196 via modem (login VISITOR). You'll find a complete listing of freenets around the world by going to NPTN Special

Projects, About the National Public Telecomputing Network (NPTN), and NPTN Affiliates and Organizing Committees.

Well-organized freenets are available in places as diverse as Youngstown, Ohio; Big Sky, Montana; Blacksburg, Virginia; Victoria, British Columbia; Denver, Colorado; and Ottawa, Ontario. In this guide, we discuss a few medical resources on freenets. Because most freenet information is local and because we don't want to choke freenets with outside traffic, we've chosen not to emphasize them. However, if you live in a city with a freenet, make it one of your first stops in your online medical search.

```
       <<<  Health Care Building  >>>
       < go health >

       1   About the Health Care Building
       2   Health Care Community Newsroom
       3   Healthy People 2000 - HEALTH PROMOTION
       4   Healthy People 2000 - HEALTH PROTECTION
       5   Healthy People 2000 - PREVENTIVE SERVICES
       6   Surveillance and Data Systems
       7   Age-related Topics - PEDIATRICS
       8   Age-Related Topics - ADOLESCENTS
       9   Age-Related Topics - SENIORS
      10   Acute or Chronic Conditions
      11   The "Health Sciences" Center
      12   Aurora Prevention Partnership
      13   Colorado Health Care Information
      14   The Support Group Center
      ----------------------------------------------
      <h>elp, <m>ain, <p>revious, <s>end mail, e<x>it DFN.

      Your Choice ==>
```

Denver Free-Net

Freenets usually offer a medical area, such as the Denver Free-Net's Health Care Building.

3
Commercial online services

With millions of Americans flocking to cyberspace, the pace of change in commercial online offerings defies any attempt to catalog what's available. In this guide, we haven't included general pricing information, but we do identify specific medical resources that might entail additional costs. Most services offer a standard monthly fee with a per-hour cost after a certain number of free hours. Some have more complicated pricing structures that vary with the time of day you call, the speed of your modem, the specific resources you want to access (often on a two- or three-tiered price schedule), and the amount of time you're online. We've provided you with toll-free numbers to contact each service for the latest details on costs and resources. Upon request, online services will also send you a startup kit.

While prices have dropped, resources have expanded. Even the medical resources we review here are only a slice of what's available. Of course, each service has dozens of other features unrelated to health. Before deciding which service to join, compare the menus of offerings. Also, consider the price and level of Internet access provided. The Internet offerings by commercial services were in a state of flux at the time this book was written.

All commercial services also offer live conferences or chat sessions that you might find informative and supportive. The format and commands of these conferences vary with each service. Some allow you to call a service representative if a participant becomes disruptive, masquerades as a healthcare professional, or spreads misinformation. Some services also archive transcripts of larger meetings at which medical experts serve as guest hosts.

In this chapter, we identify the scope of health information and the tone of support available on each commercial service. We also tell you where to find medical information after you sign on. In the next chapter, we include a sample search for information on Alzheimer's disease that demonstrates the breadth and depth of cyberspace resources, including the major commercial services, two BBSs, a freenet, and the Internet.

America Online
800-827-6364 (voice)

With a user-friendly graphical interface, America Online (AOL) is one of the easiest services to navigate, and it offers dozens of medical resources. While AOL doesn't provide access to information retrieval services, such as IQUEST or DIALOG (which also cost more), you'll find well-organized, well-managed, and well-stocked forums within AOL. You can search most forums by keyword.

– 17 –

America Online's health forums, such as HealthFocus, are easily navigated.

Inside each you'll usually find a folder with documents detailing the purpose of the forum and names of its sponsors and host. You can click on the INDEX button at the bottom of the screen to view a directory tree that shows the location of every item in the forum. Almost all forums have message centers, conference rooms, and software libraries, plus folders with informational files that, to a certain extent, make up for the lack of access to expensive commercial databases. On AOL message centers, you can read the full list of threads, including the number of messages and date of first and last posting.

America Online's Newsstand has many useful publications. Scientific American (keyword SCI AM) has a huge searchable collection of articles on biomedical topics, plus a link to the Internet. The New York Times (keyword TIMES) offers several science articles, occasional medical articles, and Jane Brody's column on health and nutrition. Consumer Reports (keyword CONSUMER REPORTS) carries a few articles about health and medicine. You can search the American Broadcasting Company (keyword ABC) for medical stories. Other online publications that you can search for medical stories include the Atlantic Monthly, the Chicago Tribune, Columnists & Features, Elle Magazine, Longevity Magazine, San Jose Mercury News, Smithsonian Publications, Time Magazine, Wired Magazine (for telemedicine updates), and Woman's Day Magazine. You can also search Today's News (keyword NEWS) for late-breaking medical stories.

In addition, you can turn to the Education Center or Reference Desk for health and medical information. In the Education Center, you'll find AskERIC, The Discovery Channel, Compton's Encyclopedia, The Learning Channel, the Library of Congress, Scientific American, Smithsonian Online, and others. The Reference Desk offers many databases you can search, including Bulletin Board Services, Health & Medical Information, and Senior Citizen Information, plus standard references you'd expect to find in your local library. The Bulletin Board Systems Corner provides a database of health-related BBSs, and the Reference Desk offers its own help section and a link to the Internet Center.

You can search Clubs & Interests by keyword, but you'll find most medical information in Health & Fitness, which we'll discuss at greater length in part two, *Where to find online medical resources.* Even Marketplace offers medical products and services in its shopping catalog. For example, members can request pharmacy deliveries to their homes. Worried about health problems on the road? Use keyword TRAVEL FORUM to read health-related travel warnings and public announcements issued by the State Department.

Internet connection

America Online's Internet Connection offers a simple on-ramp to the Internet. In addition to providing access to e-mail, mailing lists, Usenet newsgroups, gopher, WAIS, FTP, and WWW, AOL offers an online version of *Zen and the Art of the Internet*, a book about the Internet for novice users by Brendan Kehoe. Besides browsing, you can search it for answers to specific questions. America Online also has connections to the Electronic Frontier Foundation, Wired Magazine, and the PC and Mac Communication Forums. In the Electronic Frontier Foundation forum, you can follow social and legislative trends affecting the evolution of the information superhighway. The Internet Message Board helps steer you to the hot sites on the Internet and offers a place to share your experiences with others.

America Online's Internet tools are straightforward. You can select newsgroups by categories or search by keyword. If you know the complete name, you can use the Expert Add feature. Reading newsgroups is easy. You view a list of subject threads, which lists the number of messages per thread. Just double-click on notes you want to read. Posting a message is a matter of "click, write, and send." If you've been offline for a while and don't want to read hundreds or even thousands of waiting messages, start with a fresh slate by clicking on Mark All Newsgroups Read.

Since AOL's e-mail interface is so good, you might want to subscribe to mailing lists. The Internet Connection offers a searchable database of mailing lists. Each entry contains detailed instructions on how to join and leave the list, a description of the list's goals and guidelines, and keywords to identify other similar lists. If the list is also available as a newsgroup, the entry will tell you that. America Online also reminds you that mailing lists can generate a lot of mail and that you need to empty your box regularly.

Another simplified Internet tool offered by AOL is anonymous FTP. To help cut your online time, AOL maintains a list of the best FTP sites, or you can search for your own. A good use for FTP is retrieving FAQs, which you can do from a central site (rtfm.mit.edu). America Online's list of favorite sites also includes several mirrors of popular FTP sites. That means you can stay in AOL to access files from those FTP sites. This assures a good connection (often a problem with FTP) and reduces traffic at FTP sites for other users. To transfer a file from an FTP site to your hard drive, just select the file you want and then click the Download Now icon. A bar graph displays how long the transfer will take.

America Online can also take you to almost any medical gopher, either directly or indirectly, through the Health Gopher folder. The Internet Connection's graphical interface makes it easy to identify folders, text files, WAIS databases, telnet connections, images, and so on. An open book icon indicates you can do a WAIS search in whatever database is listed. You can also Search All Gophers to find information on specific folders or menus.

Health and medical resources

keyword AARP
keyword COLUMNS (Ask. Dr. Gott)
keyword CONSUMER REPORTS
keyword disABILITIES
keyword ELLE
keyword ERIC (Educational Resources Information Center)
keyword HEALTH
keyword HEALTHFOCUS
keyword HUMAN SEXUALITY
keyword IMH (issues in mental health)
keyword LIFETIME
keyword LONGEVITY
keyword NAMI (National Alliance for the Mentally Ill)
keyword NAS (National Academy of Sciences)
keyword NMSS (National Multiple Sclerosis Society)
keyword PARENTING
keyword PIN (Parents Information Network)

keyword SENIORNET
keyword UCPA (United Cerebral Palsy Associations, Inc.)
keyword WOMAN'S DAY

CompuServe

800-524-3388 (voice)

CompuServe provides a wealth of medical information and support through an easily navigated graphical interface. CompuServe is best known for its news and information gathering services, particularly those that focus on health-related topics. These services include PaperChase, IQuest Medical InfoCenter, Physician Data Query, PsycINFO, Comprehensive Core Medical Library, Health Database Plus, and Knowledge Index, all of which charge for each use. CompuServe also provides News Source USA (go NEWSUSA), U.S. News and World Report (go USNEWS), Magazine Database Plus (go MAGDB), and several other news and wire services that carry medical information. Whenever you transfer into terminal mode for a remote database search, you can capture the text to a file and thus save your entire session.

While all these powerful searching tools come at a price, it costs little to get support and help from fellow subscribers in several health forums. You can join compassionate online communities to deal with the challenges posed by cancer, diabetes, attention deficit disorder, muscular dystrophy, or any number of disabilities. All CompuServe forums are divided into seven major areas: instructions, messages, libraries, conferencing, announcements, membership directory, and options (to tailor the forum to your interests). Because CompuServe has a worldwide membership, you'll find a broader perspective than on services limited to U.S. subscribers. The forums also offer short biographical sketches of sysops and other forum personnel, including relevant experience qualifying them for their jobs.

To ensure an open, caring, and supportive environment, CompuServe sysops can and will delete messages containing personal attacks, degrading remarks, or profanity. Sysops will also lock out any forum members who harass others or fail to follow forum rules. To support information exchange among members,

CompuServe does not charge for online time spent uploading files to forum libraries. Some forums occasionally hold online focus groups to determine how to improve service.

In addition to the extensive yet expensive medical databases, you'll find many other places on CompuServe to look for medical information. For news about medical or biotechnology companies, check Fortune Magazine (go FORTUNE). If you're interested in healthcare reform, IBM and the Employee Benefit Research Institute have posted the full text and supporting documents for all major health reform proposals. As part of the basic service, you have access to the online edition of Grolier's Academic American (go ENCYCLOPEDIA), which you can search by keyword.

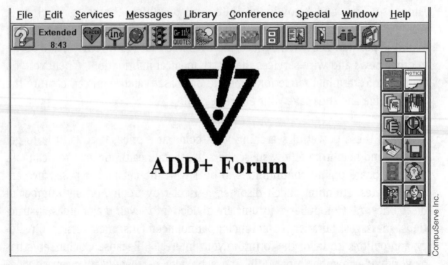

CompuServe's forums differ in appearance depending on the software used.

Internet services

CompuServe offers e-mail access to mailing lists and other Internet resources, but you'll pay extra for heavy use of e-mail services. In its Internet Services area, CompuServe offers Usenet newsgroup readers, FTP tools, and limited telnet capability. A Windows-based Web browser has also been released. For help in learning how to navigate the Internet, you can read the individual files that accompany each tool, browse Internet World Magazine articles, or join the Internet Forum.

CompuServe's Internet Services are as straightforward and utilitarian as the rest of the interface. Telnet allows you to log onto a select number of sites, including the Federal Information Exchange (see chapter 12, *Patient groups*) and the University of Minnesota Gopher Server, which gives you access to all the gophers in the world. As you'd expect, you'll find yourself in terminal emulation when using the telnet option, and you can record your session. From the Internet, you can also telnet to CompuServe to access your account.

Like America Online, CompuServe has a very simple FTP arrangement. You can select from a list of popular sites, including Ohio State University and Sunsite (both of which have many FAQs and medical files), or type in your own FTP address. CompuServe provides descriptions of popular sites so you know what to expect.

Reading Usenet newsgroups is just as easy. Start by reading what's available in a particular hierarchy (alt, misc, sci, etc.), searching by keyword, or typing in the exact name if you know it. Your newsgroup list will include the names and total number of messages for each group. When you read a newsgroup, you'll see the subject lines and number of articles per thread. You can move through a selected thread easily and either read messages online or download them to your hard drive for offline perusal. You can also specify that a file is retrieved Quoted. This means that the > symbol, used to indicate quoted online material, appears at the start of each line of the downloaded message.

Health and medical resources

go ADD (Attention Deficit Disorder Forum)
go AIDS
go APO2 (Associated Press Science & Health News)
go BIORHYTHM
go CANCER
go CCML (Comprehensive Core Medical Library)
go CNN
go COLUMNS (Her Health, His Health, The Medical Advisor)

go DIABETES
go DISABILITIES
go DRUGS (Consumer Reports Complete Drug Reference)
go ENCYCLOPEDIA (Grolier's Academic American)
go ENS (Executive News Service)
go FLATODAY (Florida Today Newslink Forum)
go GOODHEALTH (Health and Fitness Forum)
go HEALTH
go HLTDB (Health Database Plus)
go HNT (HealthNet Reference Library)
go HOLISTIC
go HRF-4794 (Sports Medicine)
go HUD (Handicapped User Database)
go HUMAN (Human Sexuality Databank and Forums)
go IBMSPECIAL (IBM Special Needs Forum)
go INFOUSA (Government Giveaways Forum)
go IQMEDICINE (IQuest Medical InfoCenter)
go ISSUES
go KI (Knowledge Index)
go MDAFORUM (Muscular Dystrophy Association Forum)
go MEDICAL
go MEDSIG (American Medical Informatics Association Forum)
go NEWAGE
go NORD (National Organization of Rare Disorders)
go NTIS (National Technical Information Service)
go PAPERCHASE
go PDQ (Physician Data Query)
go PSYCINFO (PsycINFO Database)
go RETIRE (Retirement Living Forum)
go VEGETARIAN
go WOMEN

Delphi
800-695-4005 (voice)

Delphi offers several unique features that make it an attractive place to search for and launch online medical resources. Don't be turned off by the text-based interface since you can open a log (text file) to record your entire session. If you're researching a particular medical topic, you might find a log easier than taking notes, copying text into different files, or whatever else you need to do when using a graphical interface. In addition, most assistive technology works with the Delphi text interface. The Delphi commands offer unaesthetic but powerful control over what you do online. The service provides a comprehensive manual that explains how to navigate the Delphi menu. A graphical front end for navigating the service is available for Windows users and should be ready for the Macintosh by now. If Delphi offers the information and services you want, give the service a chance.

A big selling point for Delphi is that it provides full Internet access, including e-mail, newsgroups, IRC, gopher, FTP, telnet, WWW, finger, and search tools. You can easily create your own list of favorite sites as you visit them and Delphi will automatically record the addresses. Delphi's text-based browser allows you to move through the World Wide Web quickly, although you can't view images and other graphics. For most medical searches, however, the speed of a text-based browser is worth the tradeoff.

Custom forums are another great medical resource on Delphi. You can join any custom forum at no extra charge, although some require application to the forum host. Depending on what the host decides to offer, custom forums can include a forum (message board), database, conference area, mail service, access to Usenet discussion groups and/or Internet gopher, workspace (for maintaining database files), announcements, and other special features.

Throughout part two of this book, we describe health-related custom forums and special-interest groups (SIGs). Because new custom forums are constantly being created and old ones disbanded, check Delphi to see what's currently available. You can search custom forums and SIGs by keyword (type SEARCH in the Custom Forum Directory). In addition to the medical forums listed in this section, you might want to look at Statuesque and Rubenesque (Forum 033), Animal Rights and Vegetarian Living (112), The Mommy Track (148), Cook's Corner (229), People 4 Ever (251), What's In Store (328), or Black News Network (419), among others, for more medical information.

Aside from the custom forums and Internet access, Delphi offers a few other features useful for online medical research. The Reference and Education menu lets you access the New Parents Network, CAIN (Computerized AIDS Information Network), and Grolier's Online Encyclopedia, and conduct online research with Searchline Associates, Inc. (quite expensive). We'll discuss some of these resources in the next part of the book.

> Having been diagnosed with diabetes in 1985, I know how important it is for diabetics and their family and friends to have a place to go for support. The first thing I did after my diagnosis was publish a newsletter, but postal rates were very expensive and I couldn't afford to mail newsletters to everyone who requested them.
>
> I decided to open an online support group of my own. At first I thought I would have to buy thousands of dollars worth of computer equipment and pay for expensive telephone lines.
>
> Then I logged onto Delphi Internet Services. There, much to my surprise, I discovered that Delphi would let someone like me open my own forum with access to people all over the country. Delphi also offered the lowest rates I had ever seen. Since diabetics pay for a lot of supplies and doctor visits, Delphi's low hourly rates meant I could offer an online support group other diabetics could afford.
>
> Three friends I met online (Robert Blackburn, Robert Eshelman, and Richard Eshelman) and I opened the Diabetic Friends Action Network (DFAN) forum in July of 1994. The forum includes a message section, a database, and a conference area. In the message section, anyone, diabetic or not, can leave questions that will be answered promptly. Our database contains files on different diabetes topics that members can download or read online. We also offer live conferences four nights a week. Forum members can cyber-socialize and chat. We feel it's important for people to feel comfortable. We let them know they can talk about anything in their lives, including topics other than diabetes.

The most important part of keeping a forum up and running is letting members know you appreciate their being there and participating. If no one participates, a forum is just a lifeless piece of data. Once people get involved and start sharing experiences, the board comes alive. We now send our newsletter to over 900 people each month. We no longer worry about rising postal rates since e-mailing our newsletter now takes about two seconds and costs a fraction of a penny.

We're not a huge forum, but our online family is one of the best I've ever dealt with. We have members who range in age from 10 to 70, diabetics and nondiabetics. It's quite a diverse group. I can remember one night during a live conference we were able to convince a man to start taking control of his diabetes. And there are the times when someone says to me, "I thought I was the only one who felt this way."

This makes me recognize how vital our online group is and that we're making a difference in the lives of our members.

BELVE@delphi.com

Starting your own custom forum

One reason Delphi has so many medical support groups is the ease with which users can start custom forums. The cost of maintaining a forum on Delphi goes down as usage of the forum goes up. Hosts, therefore, have a financial incentive to make the forum appealing by stocking the database with useful software and text files, scheduling live conferences, providing links to related newsgroups and gopher servers, and encouraging dynamic discussions in the message area. Forum hosts pay a start-up fee and monthly maintenance fee. If you're willing to take on this responsibility, you'll be surprised how easy and reasonably priced launching your own forum can be. Check online (go CUSTOM FORUM) for instructions and the latest pricing information.

As host, you have control over access to your forum. You can use a lock-out feature if individual members become disruptive. This is sometimes important in support groups where a cooperative atmosphere is crucial. You also control the selection of discussion topics (as many as 16 per forum), and can close certain topics to some forum members. You can edit or delete individual messages and polls, and further customize your forum by making specific Usenet newsgroups accessible to your members. You can also create and edit online banners to announce upcoming events or make recommendations about joining specific threads or reading new files.

If your forum really takes off, you can apply to expand the forum to a SIG, which means you don't have to share a database with other forums, you have access to additional Internet features, and you can establish a member directory along with other customized features. Because SIGs must follow Delphi guidelines, you have less control over the forum. Delphi encourages free and open discussion, so SIG managers step in only when absolutely necessary. Managers must also be accessible to members and work hard to keep abreast of their SIG topics. For medical groups, managers are responsible for announcing results of new studies, providing contact information for support organizations, researching and responding to member queries in the forum, and inviting medical experts to guest-host live conferences.

Internet SIG

Another important component of Delphi's medical resources is its Internet access and support. To gain Internet access, you must register and confirm that you understand Delphi isn't responsible for whatever you discover on the global network. To send and receive e-mail from the Internet, you'll need to join the Internet SIG. The Internet SIG Forum also offers a comprehensive FAQ about the Internet.

The Internet connection is quite straightforward. When you're using telnet, FTP, or IRC tools, a prompt appears, at which point you must enter an address. Delphi explains each of these features, listing the commands you need to know. Similarly, before you use finger and other Internet locator tools, Delphi offers a brief description of the resource.

Delphi also provides access to Usenet newsgroups and gopher servers. You can create your own personal list of favorites, select from a list offered by Delphi, or search by keyword (this applies to mailing lists, too). Delphi offers two ways

```
┌──────────────────────────────────────────────────────────────────┐
│ ┌──────┐ ┌──────┐ ┌──────┐ ┌──────┐ ┌──────┐ ┌──────┐ ┌──┐        │
│ │ ☀    │ │  ◈   │ │  ⬈⬋  │ │ MAIL │ │  📖  │ │OFF   │ │ ? │       │
│ │DELPHI│ │      │ │      │ │      │ │      │ │LINE  │ │   │        │
│ └──────┘ └──────┘ └──────┘ └──────┘ └──────┘ └──────┘ └──┘        │
│ Main Menu│Internet│Go To...│E-Mail│AddrBook│Log Off│Help          │
├──────────────────────────────────────────────────────────────────┤
│HEALTH AND MEDICINE                                           ▲     │
│Page 1 of 3                                                         │
│                                                                    │
│1    AIDS Information Services                       Menu           │
│2    AIDS Related Information                        Menu           │
│3    Anesthesiology Gopher (Syracuse)               Menu           │
│4    Biology subject tree                           Menu           │
│5    Biology                                        Menu           │
│6    CAMIS (Center for Advanced Medical Informatics at S  Menu     │
│7    CancerNet Information (NIH)                     Menu           │
│8    Chemistry                                      Menu           │
│9    Cornucopia of Disability Information           Menu           │
│10   Drugs                                          Menu           │
│11   Electronic Medical Journals                    Menu           │
│12   Environmental Protection Agency                Menu           │
│13   Food and Drug Administration BBS               Telnet         │
│14   Health Care Corner                             Menu           │
│15   Health Care Financing Administration           WWW/Web        │
│16   Health Sciences; L. Hancock; 03/26/94 (640K)   Text           │
│17   Health Sciences; N. Martin, P. Redman, G. Oren; 09/  Text     │
│18   Healthline gopher, U of Montana                Menu           │
│19   HSLC HealthNET                                 Telnet         │
│                                                                    │
│Enter Item Number, MORE, ?, or BACK: |                        ▼    │
├──────────────────────────────────────────────────────────────────┤
│ ◀ │                                                          │ ▶  │
└──────────────────────────────────────────────────────────────────┘
```

Delphi's Internet tools aid in researching medical topics.

of accessing Usenet newsgroups—using Delphi's own simple newsreader or a NN newsreader on a modified UNIX host. The NN has more features than Delphi's newsreader, but is harder to learn.

Delphi lists health and medicine gophers, Web sites, and telnet connections under Gopher. In addition, the top Gopher directory gives you access to more than a dozen excellent search utilities, including Archie, Veronica, WAIS, and WWW Subject Search Guides (see chapter 15, *Searching for medical resources*). The Gopher directory also provides links to several subject matter menus, which are like dynamic online yellow pages that actually do the walking to specific topics. In the Clearinghouse of Subject-Oriented Internet Resource Guides, for example, you'll find guides for alternative medicine, anesthesia and critical care, cancer, neurosciences, nursing, and women's health.

Health and medical resources

go CUSTOM 004 (Code-3)
go CUSTOM 014 (Consumer Medicine and Public Health)
go CUSTOM 015 (Handicap)
go CUSTOM 032 (Codependency Support)
go CUSTOM 046 (Nurse's Station)
go CUSTOM 065 (Yellow Submarine)
go CUSTOM 072 (Healing Place)
go CUSTOM 095 (Friends of Bill)
go CUSTOM 115 (Chronic Pain)
go CUSTOM 142 (12 Step Recovery-Sex/Love Addiction)
go CUSTOM 147 (Living Healthy)
go CUSTOM 153 (Homeopathic/Holistic Health)
go CUSTOM 169 (Respiratory Care World)
go CUSTOM 175 (Men Against Circumcision)
go CUSTOM 182 (Death & Dying Online Exchange)
go CUSTOM 215 (MS and Other Neuro-Related Disorders)
go CUSTOM 221 (Living with Brain Injury)
go CUSTOM 238 (Crohn's disease and colitis)
go CUSTOM 255 (Diabetes)
go CUSTOM 261 (Nursing Network)
go CUSTOM 264 (Child Health)
go CUSTOM 266 (Health Physics Forum)
go CUSTOM 287 (Phobias/Anxiety Support)
go CUSTOM 308 (Friends Supporting Friends)
go CUSTOM 340 (Mental Health)
go CUSTOM 351 (Depression Support Group)
go CUSTOM 355 (Multiple Personality Disorder)
go CUSTOM 377 (Nursing Student's Recovery Room)
go CUSTOM 388 (Lung Disorders)
go CUSTOM 398 (Students That Care, AIDS)
go CUSTOM 424 (Correctional Health)
go FORUM 18, U.K. Delphi (Medical Forum)
go FORUM 54, U.K. Delphi (Nursing Forum)
go GR MENSNET
go GR NEW AGE

go GR SENIORS
go GR WIDNET (World Institute on Disability Network)
go REF CAIN (Computerized AIDS Information Network)

e•World

800-775-4556 (voice)

One of the newest online services, Apple Computer's e•World, integrates some of the best features from other commercial services with a user-friendly graphical interface. You can get to health information through a few paths. From the opening e•World screen, click on the Art & Leisure Pavilion to get to Living Well, Disability Connection, Mind Garden, The Natural Connection, Transformations, and Martial Arts. The Newsstand offers UPI and USA Today. The Computing Center takes you to Madenta Communications and Straight to the Source, where you can check on several vendors that offer assistive hardware and software. Through the e•World directory, you can access Health and Fitness, Disabilities Resources, and Cooking and Nutrition. e•World, like America

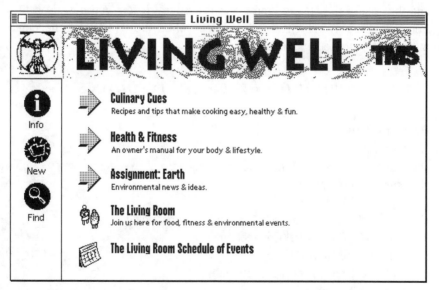

e•World offers many helpful features on its health forums, such as a new files folder and search tool.

Online, doesn't offer access to outside information searching services, such as IQUEST or DIALOG, but it does offer hundreds of well-written documents in its own forums.

You might also want to check other e•World resources for medical information, including its online multimedia encyclopedia (shortcut GROLIER). If you're looking for financial aid and other funding opportunities to help people with disabilities, search RSP Funding Focus (shortcut RSP). Nolo Press (shortcut NOLO PRESS), the leading publisher of self-help law books and software, addresses some medical-related legal issues, such as the Americans with Disabilities Act, family and medical leave, Medicaid, insurance claims, patient directives, workers' compensation, and personal injury claims. If you think laughter is the best medicine, check out the archive of lawyer jokes.

e•World forums most closely match those of America Online. Within each forum you'll find icons for new additions, general information, message boards, software and file libraries, searchable databases, live conference rooms, folders with full-text documents, and comments to forum managers. Also like America Online, e•World message boards list the number of messages in each thread and the date of the first and most recent postings. Before you download files from a library, e•World tells you the contents of the file, its size, and the length of time the download will take.

Health and medical resources

shortcut AAIN (African American Information Network)
shortcut DISABILITY
shortcut LIVING WELL
shortcut MADENTA (Madenta Communications, assistive technology)
shortcut MARTIAL ARTS
shortcut MG (Mind Garden)
shortcut STTS (Straight to the Source, assistive technology)
shortcut TNC (The Natural Connection)
shortcut TRANSFORMATIONS
shortcut UPI (United Press International)
shortcut USA TODAY

GEnie

800-638-9636 (voice)

GEnie is another text-based online service that, as you search, captures text for later viewing. The text interface is also accessible to many people with disabilities. For point-and-click navigation, you can either request by phone or download free graphical front-end programs.

GEnie organizes most medical resources into roundtables that might include bulletin boards, real-time conferences, software and document libraries, a highlighted file of the week, a newsletter, and links to related resources on GEnie. GEnie divides bulletin boards further into categories or topics of discussion. You can go to either the Medical or Disabilities RoundTable to ask health-related questions, look for medical information, or find support for dealing with a specific disease or disorder.

> My name is Dave Oberhart. In "real life" I teach courses in communications and media arts at Niagara County Community College in western New York. In my spare time, I'm also the chief sysop of an online community of wonderful people who frequent the DisAbilities RoundTable on GEnie. I have been associated with this RoundTable (RT) and GEnie for more than seven years.
>
> For disabled people, the online world offers much. I hope that on GEnie's DisAbilities RT we give a little of everything that people might find enjoyable. I've always viewed the computer and the ability to use online services as "the great equalizer." When people use a computer to communicate with others, either in a chat conference or on a bulletin board, it doesn't matter what they look like, what type of disability they might have, how old they are, or what equipment they use to access their individual systems. Everyone is playing on the same level. There are no physical barriers, no people shying away because you're in a wheelchair or because you look different. You're just someone talking to others about this or that.

– 33 –

In the DisAbilities RT, we try to offer areas for everyone to get what they need. We want people to have a place to ask questions about issues relating to disabilities. The questions might come from a family member coping with a newly diagnosed disability, an employer who has hired a disabled person, or someone with a question of a general nature—all are welcome.

Along with information, we offer a place where people with disabilities can come for support. The ability to drop by now and then to talk with people in similar situations is an invaluable service. There is much of this type of discussion in our bulletin board, along with hundreds of other disability-related topics.

I'm often asked how to describe the DisAbilities RT on GEnie. The first word that usually comes to mind is *community*. We're a large group of people with much in common, starting with our interest in issues relating to disabilities. Most of all, the people who populate the DisAbilities RT on GEnie are friendly people who like to talk, who enjoy learning new things, and who love to meet new people when they arrive.

Dave Oberhart
Chief Sysop, DisAbilities RoundTable
ABLE-DAVE@GENIE.COM

You can also look at the Public Forum RoundTable to discuss biomedical issues, 12-step programs, and issues affecting science and society. An Emergency RoundTable covers 911 topics, such as emergency assistance, first aid, cold weather hazards, and hazardous materials. This RoundTable contains information about both natural and man-made disasters anywhere in the world, and provides help in contacting people involved in a disaster. It is not, however, a place to post emergency requests for medical help.

You might find other GEnie features useful in your quest for medical information. The Research & Reference Services menu lists more than two dozen data-

```
┌─────────────────────────────────────────────────────┐
│ [─]        Medical Bulletin Board           [▼][▲]    │
├─────────────────────────────────────────────────────┤
│                    New Items                          │
│                                                       │
│  32 New Categories -- 0 New Topics -- 1167 New Messages│
├─────────────────────────────────────────────────────┤
│ [ ]📁 ASK THE DOCTOR: Specific Questions about Speci ↑ │
│ [ ]📁 Computers and Medicine                          │
│ [ ]📁 Emergency Medicine                              │
│ [ ]📁 Ear, Noise and Throat                           │
│ [ ]📁 Internal Medicine                               │
│ [ ]📁 Musculoskeletal/Orthopedic/Podiatric            │
│ [ ]📁 Neurology                                       │
│ [ ]📁 Obstetrics and Gynecology                       │
│ [ ]📁 Pediatrics                                      │
│ [ ]📁 Psychiatry/Psychology                           │
│ [ ]📁 Pulmonary                                       │
│ [ ]📁 The Nurses' Station                             │
│ [ ]📁 Paramedical Lounge (EMT, PA, RT, OT, PT, Etc.)  │
│ [ ]📁 Medical Transcriptionists                       │
│ [ ]📁 Pharmaceuticals and Drugs                       │
│ [ ]📁 Alternative Health Care                         │
│ [ ]📁 Homeopathy                                      │
│ [ ]📁 Person-to-Person Support Groups                 │
│ [ ]📁 AIDS (Support and Info)                         │
│ [ ]📁 Allergies/Asthma/Breathing (Support and Info)   │
│ [ ]📁 Alzheimers (Support and Info)                   │
│ [ ]📁 Cancer (Support and Info)                       │
│ [ ]📁 Headaches and Fibromyalgia (Support and Info)   │
│ [ ]📁 Infertility (Support and Info)                  │
│ [ ]📁 Loss and Grief (Support and Info)               │
│ [ ]📁 Pregnancy/Childbirth/Infants (Support and Info) │
│ [ ]📁 Psycotherapy (Individual/Marriage/Family)     ↓ │
└─────────────────────────────────────────────────────┘
```

GEnie's Medical RoundTable covers many health topics in one convenient location.

base services, most at an additional cost. You can access three medical research centers—AIDS Research Center, Consumer Medicine, and Medical Professional Center—all of which we review in part two, *How to find online medical resources*. GEnie offers access to DIALOG, which can be very costly. GEnie's Reference Center contains resources in more than a dozen areas of study, including medicine and psychology.

You'll also pay extra to search the Bibliographic Citations Center, which will give you a list of the most recent articles about your topic. At GEnie's Newsstand, you can search by topic, person, company, or location and retrieve full-text online articles. If you're looking for a particular book or book review, you can go to the GEnie Bookshelf to search by title, subject, author, and year. Searching both the Newsstand and the Bookshelf entail separate charges. You can then purchase books through Read USA in the GEnie Mall. Finally, you can search several online publications (at an extra cost for each), including the Los Angeles Times, Chicago Tribune, Washington Post, San Francisco Chronicle, Boston Globe, and USA Today. Detailed instructions, sample searches, and pricing information for all these services are available online.

Internet services

Before jumping onto the Net, you'll want to visit the GEnie Internet Education Center, which provides excellent Internet help. Download the Roadmap Course to learn more about using the Internet. If you're using only e-mail, you can use the center's resources to search for and download FTP files on the Internet. You can also access gopherspace via e-mail. The Internet RoundTable is extremely well organized, complete, and full of useful information. The libraries contain archived digests of Usenet newsgroups, including sci.med, plus FAQs, software, and information about using the Internet. The Internet Bulletin Board offers announcements, FAQs, and other pertinent information.

GEnie's Internet Services are straightforward and easy to use with a fingertip guide. Available Internet tools include gopher, WWW (via Lynx, a text-based browser), telnet, FTP, and Usenet newsgroups. To start exploring gopher tunnels, choose Gopher from the menu. Among the top-level choices are All the Gophers in the World, Gopher Jewels, and Veronica. You can also type in your own gopher address. GEnie explains how to use Veronica and WAIS in simple terms.

On GEnie's Web interface, hypertext links are either in color or underlined. You'll need to know at least a few commands to get around with Lynx, so be sure to take time to read the help files.

The FTP directory includes a list of individual files or collections of files and an option to type in your own FTP instructions. You'll need to use a few dreaded UNIX commands, but GEnie helps you along. Still, if you're accustomed to a graphical interface, you might be turned off by FTP services here.

GEnie's telnet menu lets you jump right into cyberspace or go to some pre-arranged sites, conveniently organized by topic. Although GEnie's newsreader didn't arrive with the other Internet goodies, it should be available now.

Health and medical resources

keyword ABLE
keyword ARC (AIDS Research Center)
keyword DIALOG
keyword MEDICAL
keyword MEDICINE (consumer medicine)
keyword MEDPRO (Medical Professional's Center)
keyword NEWAGE
keyword QUIKNEWS (news-clipping service)

Prodigy
800-776-3449 (voice)

The presence of advertisements at the bottom of the screen distinguishes Prodigy from most other commercial online services. Fortunately, the ads are relatively easy to ignore. You'll also notice a distinct difference in the organization and presentation of the service. It's most efficient to use a jump word to get where you want to go. You can also use the A-to-Z index and search by

```
╔════════════════════════════════════════════════════╗
║       PRODIGY® service - BULLETIN BOARDS            ║
╠════════════════════════════════════════════════════╣
║ Bulletin Board Blurbs                               ║
║                                                     ║
║   Health Bulletin Board                             ║
║   Here you can enhance your health by sharing    ┌──────────────┐
║   information and real experiences with others.  │Go to the Board│
║   Topics: Bodybuilding; Chiropractic;            └──────────────┘
║   Cosmetic Enhancement; Dental Care; Eye Care;     ║
║   Family Medicine; Foot Care; Herbal Medicine;     ║
║   Homeopathy; Home Remedies; Hygiene; Injuries     ║
║   and Healing; Internal Medicine; Men's Health;    ║
║   Over the Counter; Pregnancy Issues; Safety       ║
║   and Prevention; Skin Care; Sleep and Dreams;     ║
║   Sports Medicine; Stress Management; Diet and     ║
║   Nutrition; Emotional Therapy; Exercise;          ║
║   Holistic Medicine; Vitamins; Weight Control;     ║
║   Women's Health.                                  ║
║   JumpWord: Health BB              Hobbies BB [>]   ║
╚════════════════════════════════════════════════════╝
```

Prodigy lets you review health-related bulletin board offerings at a glance.

keyword (such as *health*) until you find what you need. Otherwise, you'd need to check in the Reference section to find the Multiple Sclerosis area, the Home/Family/Kids section to find the Crohn's and Colitis Forum, and the Communications section to find the Health BB.

On Prodigy, you'll find the most useful medical and health information in relatively few places. Jumping to HEALTH/FITNESS takes you to a convenient directory with links to most health resources. The articles are short and written for the health-conscious consumer. Few articles have references, but when reading a document you can usually click on the RELATED button to bring up a list of articles on similar topics. To save online reading time, you can print or copy articles in a text file on your hard drive. Until Prodigy widely offers faster modem access (14.4 Kbps or 28.8 Kbps), we also suggest you avoid viewing photographs since the process is very slow.

With few exceptions, Prodigy lumps all diseases, disorders, and other medical topics into two bulletin boards (BBs): the Health BB and the Medical Support BB, the latter of which also includes disabilities, mental illness, and other psychology topics. The hierarchy for information is BB, topics, subjects, notes, and replies. Prodigy chooses the topics and limits their number to 30 in each BB, although members can suggest new topics to the board leader. Within a specific topic, however, members can start new subjects. You can search both topic and subject lists to track down the health information you want.

Prodigy BBs have board leaders, board specialists, and member representatives. Board leaders inform members about upcoming events on the board, administer topics, participate in discussions, and answer mail. Board specialists process all notes that are submitted. On the opening BB screen, you can use the ALERT mailbox to let board specialists know about problem notes. The member representative, someone who has demonstrated ongoing contributions to the board, participates in board discussions and helps other members understand how the board functions.

The Medical Support Bulletin Board (MSBB) is uniquely set apart from others on Prodigy by its personal and supportive atmosphere. Members meet here to share personal thoughts, struggles, failures, and triumphs they face with illness, disease, disabilities, or other medical conditions. Some members share daily concerns they face while caring for a family member or friend who is ill, disabled . . . even dying. They might find a listening ear, outstretched hand, or willing conversationalist to connect with on one of many topics.

Besides support, we often find opinions, information, experience, or new media news items posted by members who are researching, studying, or practicing in the field of medicine. Members, of course, are reminded in the guidelines that they must never use the information posted as their means of treatment or diagnosis, and to always consult their physician or healthcare provider.

We do have a few online specialists taking questions from members regarding illnesses or topics such as lupus, diabetes, physical therapy, urology, and obstetrics and gynecology. Guests often give online advice and suggestions to members. Upcoming guests will discuss autism, Alzheimer's disease, cancer, depression, obsessive-compulsive disorder, hemochromatosis, nuclear medicine, care-giving, attention deficit disorder, dieting, and much more.

To enhance the Medical Support BB, I added a live weekly guest program. On Wednesday nights at 8:30 p.m. (EST), the "doors open" to the Medical Support Auditorium in the Chat area of Prodigy. Each week we feature a new guest and topic.

We hope members will feel comfortable joining us on the Medical Support BB and in our Chat area, with its several Medical Support rooms. The support and warmth our board provides reaches across the country and is available daily by computer and modem. In fact, we offer a global view by providing directions to areas of medical interest on the World Wide Web. We have something for everyone. If new members don't find what they need, one of our special contributors or mem reps or I will be glad to help as best we can.

Nancy Eggleston
Prodigy Medical Support BB

On Prodigy, you can Ask Beth (jump ASK BETH) questions about parent-teenage relationships and adolescent health concerns, such as pregnancy, drug and alcohol abuse, and eating disorders. If you're considering a career in a medical field, you can jump CAREER BB to learn about admission requirements, job training, skills, and job descriptions. You can also inquire about scholarships and financial aid.

Internet Forum

Prodigy's best source of medical information is through its Internet connection. You have access to e-mail, newsgroups, and, with Windows, the World Wide Web (plus gopher and FTP throughout the Web). The star of Prodigy's Internet connection is its Usenet newsgroup interface. You can easily subscribe to newsgroups, which you'll find simply by selecting their names from a list or searching by keyword. Reading newsgroups is just as straightforward. The window lists articles by subject line with the number of messages included for each thread. You can download messages without reading them online, and search for a particular topic or author. Best of all, you can search for the newsgroup's

FAQ—the most important posting to read. If the FAQ comes in multiple parts, you can select whichever part you want to read.

The Prodigy Web browser is slow but fully functional. If you're familiar with Netscape, you'll immediately know how to use the Prodigy browser. You can create a "hot list" of favorite sites, navigate the Web easily, and tailor the browser to look the way you want. Prodigy offers online help for both the WWW and the browser.

Health and medical resources

jump AARP
jump AP ONLINE
jump CONSUMER REPORTS
jump CROHNS
jump FOOD BB
jump HEALTH BB
jump HEALTH/FITNESS
jump HEALTH NEWS
jump HEALTH TOPICS
jump KEEPING FIT
jump MEDICAL SUPPORT BB
jump MS (National Multiple Sclerosis Society)
jump NEW AGE
jump SELF
jump WOMEN

4

Sample search for online medical information

*I*magine that your mother has recently become fatigued and moody. She had been doing well despite living alone for five years after your father's death, but lately forgets your children's names. Sometimes she doesn't even recognize them. Her bank statement is a mess. She often repeats a question you just answered. Concerned about her health, you take her for a check-up. After an exam and a battery of tests, her doctor tells you the news—your mother has Alzheimer's disease.

First comes denial. She's just feeling her age, the loss of her husband. You don't want to accept she has what her doctor calls a *progressive disease*, one that will get worse over time. You feel powerless, unable to change what you fear will be a relentless downhill course.

Your mother's doctor is helpful. She recommends learning as much as you can about how the disease affects both the patient and caregiver. She also suggests you talk to a lawyer about becoming a guardian should your mother be unable to handle her own affairs. The physician gives you a pamphlet about Alzheimer's, suggests a few books to read, and urges you to join a support group. You still can't believe what's happening.

You leave the physician's office in tears. After getting over the initial shock and denial, you decide to create an action plan. That helps you feel more in control. You make phone calls. You read the materials you have. You turn your computer on. . . .

America Online

What you like best about America Online is that you can search by keyword almost every resource that offers information about Alzheimer's, and the keyword search doesn't cost extra. Although you can't access MEDLINE, which indexes most medical journals in the world, you find brief news updates, fact sheets, resource lists, long feature articles from several publications, and support from other people dealing with Alzheimer's disease. It's easy to download selected files to your hard drive. You decide to explore AOL section by section.

go ABC The American Broadcasting Company offers only a few odd snippets about Alzheimer's disease, including coverage of Ronald Reagan's condition.

go AARP Using *Alzheimer* as a keyword at the American Association of Retired Persons (AARP) forum, you find 9 matches, including 3 about caregiving. One article offers tips for coping. Another discusses a personal approach to caregiving and includes an offer for free AARP publications. There's also a document about how depression can either mimic Alzheimer's disease or be a separate feature of the disease. Other articles cover estrogen, hearing loss, long-term care insurance, a White House conference on aging and health care, and a new eye test for diagnosing the disease.

go COLUMNIST In the Lifestyles folder you find Ask Dr. Gott, which has one column about memory loss and aging. Dr. Gott also talks about Alzheimer's symptoms, provides general information about the disease, and discusses Tacrine as a possible treatment. In addition, you can order a health report about the disease.

go COMPTONS In the online encyclopedia, you find short articles about Alzheimer's disease, memory loss, and the nervous system. Unfortunately, you find no hypertext links to related topics.

America Online's American Association of Retired Persons forum can be quickly searched.

go HEALTH A keyword search of the Better Health & Medical Forum turns up 13 documents on Alzheimer's disease, including an extensive overview of the disease that answers many of your questions. There's also an article on head injury and genetic susceptibility as risk factors for Alzheimer's. The article cites an *Annals of Neurology* paper, which you note.

go HEALTHFOCUS A check of HealthFocus archives reveals several documents about Alzheimer's, including information about death and dying issues and patient care directives. There are also quizzes, tips, and a directory full of text and multimedia documents about Alzheimer's disease.

go LONGEVITY A search of the Longevity archives with the term *Alzheimer* returns 36 possibilities with several documents about coping with aging parents. One article describes how to diagnose Alzheimer's and how to rule out other disorders.

go NAS At the National Academy of Sciences, there's a reference to a new book from the Institute of Medicine entitled *Discovering the Brain*, which includes a chapter on Alzheimer's disease. Four other matches don't offer much useful information.

go SAN JOSE In the San Jose Mercury News archives, there are 10 articles about Alzheimer's disease, including one about using therapeutic art lessons to help Alzheimer's patients communicate. Another article describes a San Diego obstetrician who practiced for as many as four years while afflicted with the disease.

go SCI AM In Scientific American, your search turns up 6 articles addressing everything from genetic testing for Alzheimer's to a reduced incidence of the disease in extremely old people. There's also a feature story about new techniques for diagnosing and monitoring the progress of the disease.

go SENIORNET You've found a lot of information so far, but you're overjoyed to locate a compassionate community of people concerned about the disease. The SeniorNet forum offers discussions of long-term care with many threads offering support, resources, and sage advice. You see threads entitled Overwhelmed, Adjusting, and My Experience. You discover that two nurses offer help on the forum.

go TIME Many of the 26 matches to the term *Alzheimer* in Time magazine are brief health reports and book reviews. Other matches cover issues of aging and Alzheimer's, including how Japanese families care for older parents. You again find information about Ronald Reagan's struggle with Alzheimer's disease and a new eye test for diagnosing the disease.

go TIMES Although none of the current New York Times offerings pertain to Alzheimer's, you note that the Science Times section covers health and medicine extensively. You make a mental note to check here again for new articles.

CompuServe

Although some of the best features are costly, CompuServe has much to offer, including a lot of support and information. Since you're using the CompuServe Information Manager, you like the option of putting the most important resources in your Favorite Places list for quick access.

go CCML Your keyword search of the Comprehensive Core Medical Library for the terms *Alzheimer* and *caregiver* turns up 29 items, and you can view the most recent 10 items for $5. Some references are repeated in this first list of 10, and most are more than a year old. You pass on viewing any more items ($5 per additional 10) or on viewing the abstracts or full text of any of your current matches ($5 each). The total cost is $5 (1 successful search).

go ENCYCLOPEDIA Here a keyword search yields what you'd expect from an encyclopedia (in this case, the Academic American Encyclopedia): a short background article with links to related terms, such as neurotransmitter, acetylcholine, serotonin, and positron emission tomography.

go FLATODAY In the Florida Today Forum, an extended service, you find an article reviewing Alzheimer's disease with specific statistics and resources for Floridians.

go GOODHEALTH In the library of the Health and Fitness Forum, another extended service, you find and download the transcript of a 1992 Elder Care conference in which participants discuss the pain and frustration of caring for aging parents, including those with Alzheimer's.

go HLTDB At Health Database Plus, the search term *Alzheimer* turns up 800 references, 764 of which are distributed among 55 subdivisions. Subdivisions include Abnormal Physiology, Moral and Ethical Aspects, Prognosis, and Complications. Because your major decisions involve the care of your mother, you look under Care and Treatment and find 100 references. To cut costs, you decide to do more research elsewhere until you can run a more focused search here. The total cost is $4.50 (5 minutes of connect time and 3 full-text articles).

go HNT At HealthNet you find a comprehensive summary of Alzheimer's disease, including diagnosis, cause, treatment, prognosis, and other causes of dementia. The summary explains the medical terms in plain English.

go IUS-5996 At this extended service option, the Free Health Information and Care directory leads you to Free Information From A–Z, which has a number of listings for Alzheimer's disease. Among the offerings, you find a document with information about four clearinghouses/hotlines, a list of (and ordering information for) free publications and videos about Alzheimer's disease, and a list of free docu-

Sample search for online medical information

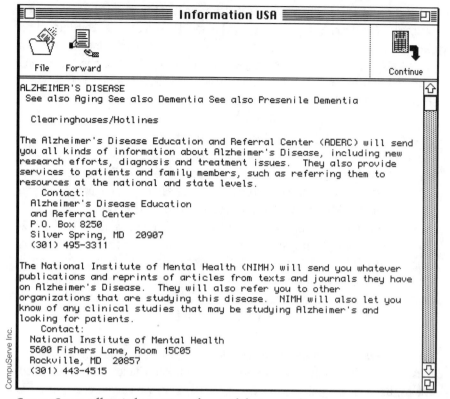

CompuServe offers information about Alzheimer's disease, for example, at *Information USA*.

ments from various government agencies (phone numbers, document numbers, and descriptions included).

go IQMEDICINE In the Medicine & Allied Health menu, you scan the Consumer Health databases. Using *Alzheimer* and *caregiver* as search terms, you go ahead with the $5 scan that retrieves references from five databases: Ageline, Allied & Alternative Medicine, Family Resources, Magazine ASAP, and Magazine Index. The Family Resources database has 35 references, all of which you decide to view. Fortunately, IQUEST keeps you abreast of your charges as you go. You'll have to pay $9 to view the first 10 references and $9 for each additional 10 references, with an additional $3 per abstract. Full-text reprints cost $18 (regular mail) or $42 (express mail). In the Allied & Alternative Medicine database, it will cost

$11 to view five matching references that are similar to those you've seen in other databases. You decline to pay more for the additional materials. You then check the first 10 references you retrieved from the Family Resources database and find that all references are more than a year old. You decide not to check any more matches in this or any other Consumer Health database. The total cost is $30 (2 successful scans and 2 successful searches).

go KI You head to Knowledge Index to search the DIALOG databases. The first search with just the keyword *Alzheimer* produces 12,376 records. Adding the keyword *caregiver* reduces the number of records to 147. To ensure you have only the latest information, you further limit the search to the current and prior years. That cuts the list to 30. To eliminate animal or foreign studies, you narrow the search to human and English-language articles. That brings the list down to 29 articles, which you then display. Two look promising, but one, a letter from Lancet, is not full text. You read an abstract from a *Journal of Gerontology* article about self-control skills among caregivers. To avoid additional costs, you decide to examine the rest of the list offline before requesting more references. You log off. The total cost is $1.80 (for more than 6 minutes of connect time).

go MAGDB Although each search adds more expense, you check Magazine Database Plus. Your search on *Alzheimer* turns up 228 citations, 226 in 28 subdivisions, but you find only 15 in Care and Treatment, which you check first. The articles come from such diverse sources as *Family Circle*, *Scientific American*, *The Economist*, and *Good Housekeeping*, with some articles duplicating the Health Database Plus search. You read the full text of two articles, one from *People* magazine on caregiving and the other from *Aging* entitled "Difficult Decisions: A Family Deals with Alzheimer's Disease." The total cost is $3 (4 minutes of connect time and 2 full-text articles).

go MEDSIG You check out another extended service, the American Medical Informatics Association Forum, where you search the library's alphabetical index for Alzheimer's files. You download one file of references on the relationship between smoking and Alzheimer's disease. Your mother smoked, so you skim the available abstracts.

Sample search for online medical information

go NORD Although Alzheimer's isn't a rare disease, you search another extended services option, the NORD (National Organization of Rare Diseases) database. You find an overview of Alzheimer's, its symptoms and causes, the affected population, and standard and investigational therapies. You also check a list of resources and references. Of these, the most interesting are investigational therapy pages describing clinical studies of drugs to treat the disease.

go NTIS You decide to search the National Technical Information Service. Using the term *Alzheimer*, you find 8 items, 2 of which you decide to view. One is about biomedical features of Alzheimer's, and the other is about brain destruction and aluminum accumulation. While both are interesting, neither is particularly useful. The items you didn't view are even more scientific in nature. The total cost is $9 (1 search and 2 abstracts).

go PAPERCHASE Using PaperChase to access the National Library of Medicine's MEDLINE, Health, AIDSLINE, and CANCERLIT databases, you can select subject keywords, author's name, journal title, or institutional address to define your search. Your choice of *Alzheimer's disease* turns up 12,020 matches. To help narrow the search, the program offers a long list of subheadings. You choose *rehabilitation*, which drops the number of matches to 63. As you read the citations in the list, most are identified as [NO ABSTRACT ONLINE]. This helps you limit your viewing to the three citations with an online abstract, thus saving you time and money. After you log off, you conclude that PaperChase offers the cheapest commercial option for searching for medical articles. The total cost is $1.66 (5.53 minutes at $18 an hour).

go PEOPLE A search of *People* magazine archives yields 6 citations, including an article about how Nancy and Ronald Reagan are dealing with the former President's condition. The total cost is $1.50 (2 minutes of connect time and 1 full-text article).

go RETIRE Another extended service option, the Retirement Living Forum offers a health and medical library and message section where you find a long Alzheimer's thread. In the discussion, members talk about everything from nicotine patches to Cognex. A pharmacist even volunteers information about specific drugs and their side effects. You download an article by Safe Technologies

Corporation about a possible link between electromagnetic fields and Alzheimer's disease. In the Family and Aging section, another Alzheimer's thread offers advice from caregivers and health professionals around the world. Discussion ranges from day care to durable power of attorney.

goUSNEWS A search of back issues of U.S. News and World Report yields 13 full-text articles, 2 of which you download (one on new diagnostic tests, the other on a new theory about how the disease progresses). The total cost is $3 (3 minutes of connect time and 2 full-text articles).

Delphi

A look at the opening menus offers no clues on where to search. The news isn't organized by health topics, and the Senior Forum is barren. You find little in a search of the custom forums for information on *Alzheimer's, caregiver,* and *aging.* Ditto for the Nursing Network Forum. At least custom forums 308 (Stress-Free Support and MS) and 215 (Other Neuro-Related Disorders) offer places to talk with others, and you apply to join them. To find information on Alzheimer's, you realize you need to bypass the rest of Delphi and head for the Internet area.

go CUSTOM 014 You're disappointed to discover that the Public Health Forum has nothing in its database that matches the terms *Alzheimer's, caregiving,* or *aging.* When you search the forum's message subject lines for *Alzheimer,* you find three old postings about starting an Alzheimer's support group but nothing further. You write down the e-mail addresses of the two people involved. The Usenet discussion groups have nothing to suit your needs.

go INTERNET Before launching your Internet research (the details are given later in this section), you decide to choose the option Search All Usenet FAQs (Swiss source) to look for Alzheimer's information. An article about tinnitus, or ringing in the ear, is the only match. Using Search All Usenet FAQs (Swedish source), you find the Cryonics FAQ, which says Alzheimer's patients shouldn't bother going through the freeze-dried process to wait for a cure. Memory loss will probably never be restored.

go REF GROLIER At Delphi's online encyclopedia, a search for *Alzheimer*
yields one brief article with a bibliography.

e•World

Despite its entertaining interface, e•World offers little useful information.
There's no discussion of Alzheimer's disease in the health-related forums. A
keyword search of Living Well produces nothing for *Alzheimer* and only a few
matches for *aging*, including a pamphlet offered by the Family Doctor.

shortcut DISABILITY You go to the Disability Connection to search ABLEDA-
TA (in the Research Headquarters) for Alzheimer's-related assistive technology. You
get information on 7 products, including special beds, air support systems, and
monitoring devices to prevent wandering. Two monitoring systems sound especially useful. You also notice with interest and a bit of sadness an entry for a Discovery
Apron, designed for people with Alzheimer's to keep their hands purposefully
occupied with familiar objects or actions like zippers, pockets, and materials with
different textures.

shortcut GROLIER Your keyword search of *Alzheimer* on e•World's online
encyclopedia turns up articles on aluminum, Alzheimer's disease, Sir Rudolf Bing,
Down's syndrome, geriatrics, hospital, mental disorder, diseases of the nervous system, psychopathology, radiology, senility, taste and smell, and, of all things, Joanne
Woodward (no, she doesn't have Alzheimer's disease—she portrayed a patient).

shortcut NOLO PRESS Your search for medical topics in the main e•World
directory suggests Nolo Press. The keyword *Alzheimer* refers you to information
about the Family and Medical Leave Act and how to beat the "insurance racket."

shortcut TRANSFORMATIONS At first, Transformations looks appealing,
but there's no keyword search service so you must look through folders individual-
ly. One vaguely titled document, Elderly, is a great source of contacts and background information on Alzheimer's and other disorders in older adults, but on the
Medical Support Groups bulletin board you find almost no discussion in the

– 51 –

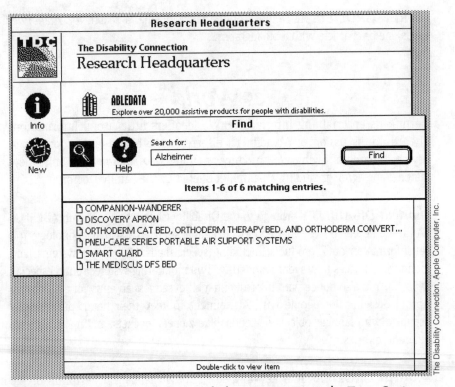

e•World's Disability Connection includes ABLEDATA at the Trace Center Cooperative Library.

Caregivers Support thread. You recognize that the forum is new, and hope to find more here later.

shortcut UPI A search of UPI news for *Alzheimer* produces a one-paragraph story on Canadian research for a new drug that reverses memory deficits in aged animals. You also find an article that says it costs a frightening $33,000 annually to care for someone with Alzheimer's disease.

GEnie

Searching for information in GEnie is easy but generally expensive. You can keep track of your running total and are warned when your next choice will be expensive. There's also a wonderful support group available.

Sample search for online medical information

keyword ARC Remembering that dementia often occurs in AIDS, you decide to check the AIDS Research Center for more information. Here Alzheimer produces 81 matches, 10 of which you view. You read the abstract of one article comparing AIDS and Alzheimer caregivers and their use of computer networks for support. The total cost is $6 (1 search, 10 records listed, and 1 record viewed).

keyword DIALOG Having checked on CompuServe's Knowledge Index DIALOG resources, you decide to see what GEnie's DIALOG connection has to offer. Working through the menus to the Health area, you run an *Alzheimer* search ($2.50) and find 4,778 articles. You add *caregiver* to the list of search terms and focus by year (1994–1995). This brings the total to $5, but cuts the choices down to 14. You decide to list all 14 records and view 4 of them (2 citations, 1 abstract, and 1 full-text article about depression and anxiety among Alzheimer caregivers). The article is informative, but you're not sure you'll hurry back to DIALOG again because of the cost. The total cost is $36.50 (2 searches, 14 records listed, and 4 records viewed).

keyword MEDICAL At the Medical RoundTable (which is thankfully free), you search the libraries first and find 7 files, including a document from the FDA about Tacrine, several medical newsletter updates, and transcripts of past Alzheimer's meetings. You then search all bulletin board categories for Alzheimer and find Caregivers for Alzheimer's Disease in the Person-to-Person Support Groups category. It's described as "a place for Alzheimer's caregivers to share the frustration, ideas, and experiences of everyday living with others whose lives have been changed and controlled by this dread disease." You notice that group members generously support one another. You also find a separate category for Alzheimer Support and Information, where you read many helpful, compassionate messages.

keyword MEDICINE You decide to use the Consumer Medicine premium service to thoroughly search the available literature. A search using the keyword *Alzheimer* brings up 8,675 records, 10 of which are listed (running bill: $3). Adding *caregiver* as another search term cuts the list to 31 records, with 10 shown ($6). Viewing the remaining 21 records brings the bill to $15 and reveals an article about online support for Alzheimer's caregivers. Interested in this subject, you're disappointed to find only the citation and a not very informative abstract. The total cost is $18 (2 searches, 31 records listed, and 1 record viewed).

keyword MEDPRO You try another premium service, Medical Professional's Center, to see if you can find anything else in the medical literature. This time the Alzheimer search turns up 36,273 records in 10 databases ($2.50). The database carries the full text of the *New England Journal of Medicine.* You decide to check 50 citations from this prestigious journal (the first 10 are shown, at a running cost of $7.00). Included are book reviews, letters, images, research articles, review articles, and special reports. Although you were warned of the cost in advance, you decide to list all 50 citations (for an additional $18). You elect to view the full text of one article, a double-blind, controlled trial of Tacrine. The total cost is $29.50 (1 search, 50 records listed, and 1 record viewed).

keyword REFCENTER A check of the GEnie Reference Center for *Alzheimer* yields 34,064 records in 16 databases, including Art, Philosophy, World History, Agriculture, and Engineering. Adding the keyword *caregiver* narrows the list to 131 choices in 6 databases: Medicine, Psychology, Biology, Sociology, Education, and Popular Magazines. You opt to read the full text of one Popular Magazine article that examines the impact on the immune system of a caretaker whose relative has Alzheimer's. A check of the first 10 of 38 records in the Medicine database yields titles that you've seen in previous searches. The same is true for the Psychology database, where you list 10 of 37 records. The total cost is $23 (2 searches, 22 records listed, and 1 record viewed).

Prodigy

A search for Alzheimer's disease resources on Prodigy yields some support resources, but little information compared with the other online services.

jump AARP With no way to search the forum, you go through promising menu options but find nothing on Alzheimer's disease. The Home/Family section offers a general document with tips for caregivers, but no mention of Alzheimer's.

jump HEALTH There's nothing related to aging or Alzheimer's in the topic list. You check the Other topic list and find an Alzheimer subject with a note from one person asking for help. The reply to the note refers the person to the Medical Support BB, which is where you now head.

jump MED SUPPORT You look through the topics of the Medical Support BB and find several promising leads under both Caregivers and Alzheimer's. Under the topic Caregivers you find useful postings in subjects entitled Caregiving Newsletter, Financial Info, Nursing Homes, and Aging Parent/Child. As you read through the last subject, you're amazed at how many other people share your situation. Under the topic Alzheimer's you find a posting from a woman who has cared for her mother for six years. Another posting warns about side effects of medications. Another offers a perspective on handling parents in the early stage of the disease. Titles of messages include Oh God What To Do, It's Over, Just Beginning, and Strength To Go On. It's encouraging that newcomers to the group receive compassionate replies from other members, who seem very familiar with one another.

Bulletin board systems
Black Bag BBS
610-454-7396

First you go to the Bulletin menu where you select Info for the Elderly, which explains the disease and treatment options. You move through the menus until you get to Medbase. You go to the Problems/Disorders directory, then to the Neurological/Muscular menu, and then to the Alzheimer's file. Here a document in outline format summarizes the disease. You locate other Alzheimer's files that cover the disease itself, Alzheimer's-related depression, head trauma, and patient characteristics at each stage of the disease. You then go to the message area and decide to join groups with an international reach—Alzheimer's Discussion (#A97), Care Giver Support Echo (#68), Ask A Nurse National Echo (#53), and Grand Rounds Medical Echo (#13).

AgeNet
800-989-2243

Although AgeNet is designed for use by people who develop and provide services for older adults, the BBS provides access to some useful databases. The Information and Referral Bibliography database offers descriptions and contact information for 24 Alzheimer's resources, ranging from programs to books to videos. Two other databases, Connections and Skills, provide names of additional contacts and services.

Freenet
Alzheimer's Information Center
303-270-4865, telnet freenet.hsc.colorado.edu
(login GUEST, go ALZHEIMER)

After many unsuccessful attempts, you finally log onto the Denver Free-Net and go to the Alzheimer's disease section. Here you find an Alzheimer's FAQ, which provides comprehensive background information about the disease, recommended reading, a glossary, and directions for contacting the Alzheimer's Association. There's also a listing of offline groups, mainly in the Denver area. The Legal Considerations file is excellent but focused mainly on Colorado laws. A document called Directions in Alzheimer's Research concisely reviews current efforts. The Care Planning in Nursing Homes file offers suggestions for assessing nursing homes and developing care plans.

The Internet

A couple of quick Internet searches turn up hundreds of possibilities. One title search through gopherspace alone brings 201 documents, images, and menus dealing with Alzheimer's disease. A very focused Web search to weed out the many research and scientific resources comes up with three good hits.

Alzheimer Society of Ottawa-Carleton
http://www.ncf.carleton.ca/go.html (select Alzheimer)

You hit the jackpot using the WWW to access the National Capital Freenet in Ottawa, Canada. Here the Alzheimer Society of Ottawa-Carleton has an extensive menu of useful choices. In the Public Discussion of AD directory, you find several impressive documents explaining Alzheimer's and physician guidelines for diagnosing the disease. You also check three Alzheimer Society of Canada information sheets, all of which are excellent: Risk Factors for Alzheimer Disease, Predictive Testing for Alzheimer Disease, and Alzheimer Disease and Heredity. You move to Family and Caregiver Support and find tips for traveling with an Alzheimer's patient, legal and tax issues (with a Canadian focus), assistive devices specifically for individuals with Alzheimer's, and practical considerations for the caregiver. There's also a Wandering Persons Registry, which discusses causes of wandering. A file in the Memory Disorder Clinics directory offers help in distinguishing normal forgetfulness from Alzheimer's, tips for helping the Alzheimer's patient maintain memory skills, and a list of Canadian drug trials. The Drugs in Development directory lists U.S. efforts and provides contact information.

At this site you also find resource lists and guidelines for caregiving, a news update for Alzheimer's programs and research in the United States, and an extensive list of conferences and other Alzheimer's events. There are fact sheets and other background information from Alzheimer's Disease International and a list of 28 Alzheimer's Disease Research Centers in the United States with contact information. Also available are several lists of Internet resources on neurosciences and aging in addition to a guide to Alzheimer's and other geriatric online resources. This last guide includes mailing lists, e-mail forums, Usenet newsgroups, gopher servers, Web pages, freenets, BBSs, and commercial online services.

Alzheimer Web
http://werple.mira.net.au/~dhs/ad.html

From Canada you jump to Australia, where the Alzheimer Web Home Page offers answers to general questions about Alzheimer's disease, with a special emphasis on scientific aspects. Graphics show how Alzheimer's affects the

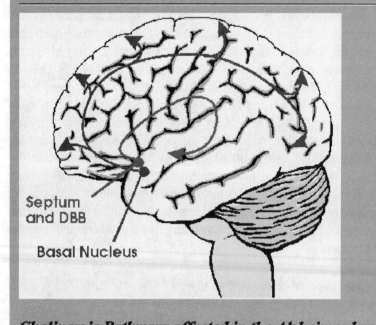

Alzheimer Web is useful for health professionals and the public.

brain. With special software you can view an MRI movie of an Alzheimer patient's brain. You also see many articles you found on commercial services, such as the *Time* magazine story about Ronald Reagan.

At the Australian site you find links to other Alzheimer's researchers, mainly in the United States, in addition to several databases and lists of medical journal articles about Alzheimer's disease. You find a link to MEDLINE, but a keyword search for *Alzheimer* and *caregiver* produces no matches. However, a search for *Alzheimer* alone produces hundreds of citations, some of which might interest your mother's physician.

You also note that this Web page is well integrated with the rest of the Internet, with direct links to a search engine, neuroscience guides (providing their own links), biochemistry and molecular biology resources, other Alzheimer's Web pages (research-oriented), and many other medical WWW sites. The page has an announcement of a new newsgroup, bionet.neuroscience.amyloid. You also notice a telnet connection back to the Alzheimer Society of Ottawa-Carleton and the opportunity to subscribe to several research-oriented mailing lists, including Amyloid, GeriNet, and Alzheimer, the latter of which is geared to a more varied audience.

Alzheimer

majordomo@wubios.wustl.edu

You then subscribe to the Alzheimer mailing list, which connects you with physicians and Alzheimer's researchers around the world. The first digest arrives with long, thoughtful messages from a physician in the United Kingdom, the research librarian at the Philadelphia Geriatric Center (posting useful information about online Alzheimer's resources), a physician from the University of California, San Diego's Alzheimer's Disease Research Center, a nurse specializing in gerontology and Alzheimer's, and Italian researchers organizing the 5th Alzheimer Europe annual meeting. Dozens of other big-hearted list members share wisdom they've gained through their experiences with Alzheimer's. You also read about the therapeutic use of animals (dogs, cats, fish, bunnies) and music. You learn that sprinkling sugar on food sometimes induces an Alzheimer's patient to eat. You read discussions about caretakers' hard decisions to move Alzheimer's patients to nursing homes. When you check the dates and times of the various postings, you realize this international discussion goes on day and night.

UnCover at CARL Corporation

telnet database.carl.org

After realizing the expense of literature searches on other commercial services, you decide to try UnCover at CARL Corporation. Initially you don't set up an account, although you'll consider it if you decide later to retrieve full-text documents. With a keyword of *Alzheimer's disease*, your first search yields 2,498 items. Adding the word *caregiver* shortens the list to 17 items, which you ask

UnCover to display. The list includes the author, publication name and date, and document title. When you ask to view an item, you're given the full author list, complete title and bibliographic references, number of pages, and summary of the document's content. UnCover notes when an article might be available for free at a local library. The service also lists fax charges. For example, ordering a fax of a recent article from the *Journal of Gerontological Nursing* on managing Alzheimer's patients at home would cost $10.75 (an $8.50 service charge and $2.25 copyright fee). You're excited about finding this free searching service and decide to telnet to CARL the next time you want to check for available literature.

5

General health information

Wouldn't it be great to have a medical encyclopedia at your fingertips? You do. It's your online connection to the Internet, commercial services, and a vast array of bulletin board systems (BBSs).

If you're looking for general information on a health topic, remedies for a cold, or advice about how often to have your blood pressure checked, you'll find answers on the Internet, either on the World Wide Web or in one of several gophers. Of course, you don't need the Internet to find a wide range of health information. Several excellent BBSs offer documents, software, and message boards to help with your medical questions. Dr. Ed Del Grosso, who maintains the Black Bag BBS, offers a list of hundreds of other health-related BBSs around the world. If you don't want to pay long-distance charges, try the National Institutes of Health (NIH) Information Center.

Finally, several commercial online services offer access to databases, reference libraries, journals, periodicals, newspapers, and wire services that will answer many of your medical questions. You can retrieve some information at standard hourly connection rates, while more thorough searches are costly.

Arizona Health Sciences Library

http://amber.medlib.arizona.edu/ahsc-res.html

Many online medical and health libraries offer little more than a slim listing of card catalogs. That's not the case with the Arizona Health Sciences Library, a full-service online resource. This site lists not only its own holdings but also gives you access to hundreds of documents, programs, and links to other online services. Useful features of the Library include answers to commonly asked health questions, health tips, and medical news releases from the University of Arizona Health Sciences Center. You'll also find a series of Web maps for nutrition, public health, and smoking cessation. Other guides geared more toward health professionals than patients include a Pediatric Critical Care Page, PathPICS (pathology images), RadPICS (radiology images), and the Grant Guide to Funding Information. While you might not want to make this site your very first stop, it's definitely worth checking out.

Black Bag BBS

610-454-7396

If you're hungry for medical information, one of the first places to call is the Black Bag BBS. You'll get a taste for using BBSs and an appreciation for the range of medical information available from your desktop. The Black Bag BBS sysop, Edward Del Grosso, M.D., maintains a list of most (if not all) of the medical, fire/EMS, science, addiction recovery, AIDS, and disability-related BBSs in the United States and Canada, in addition to many international systems. Dr. Del Grosso has operated the Black Bag BBS for more than nine years. To get a copy of the current medical BBS list, send e-mail to list@blackbag.com, or, better yet, sign on to Black Bag BBS. The following is a listing of Black Bag BBS message areas:

12 Steps to Recovery	Amputee Support Echo
AA Discussion Group	Animal Medicine
Alcoholic Families	Anxiety National Conference
Alcoholism—Drug Abuse Echo	Ask A Nurse National Echo
American Sign Language Discussion	Astronomy National Echo

Attention Deficit Disorder	Multiple Sclerosis Echo
Bicycling Forum	Narcotics Anonymous
Biomedical Conference	National Dieting Echo
Black Bag Local Chatter	National Federation for the Blind
Blind Talk	National Nutrition Talk
Blind Users National Echo	National Physics Echo
Cancer Discussion	National Psychiatry Echo
Care Giver Support Echo	Nurses Network
Cerebral Palsy Discussion	Offline Readers Support Echo
Child Abuse National Discussion	Optometry Discussion
Chronic Fatigue Syndrome	Overeaters National Echo
Chronic Pain National Echo	Physical Fitness Discussion
CVA/Stroke National Echo	Post Polio Discussion
Deaf Users Echo	Problem Child National Discussion
Diabetes National Discussion	Psychology Discussion
Disabled Athletes Discussion	Radiology Echo
Disabled National Echo	Rare Conditions National Echo
Disaster Info/Relief/Recovery	Recovery from Sexual Addiction
EmergNet Operations & Mission	Science and Technology Echo
EMS National Discussion	Science National Echomail
Fibromyalgia National Discussion	Seizure Disorders
Fire National Echomail	Social Services National Echo
Grand Rounds—Medical Echo	Spinal Injury National Discussion
Healing Via Touch	Stress Management Conference
Herb Talk	Survivors of Child Abuse Echo
Incest Survivors Conference	Survivors of Ritual Abuse
Mental Health Echo	Terminal Illness Discussion
Multipersonality Disorders Help	Therapist National Discussion
Multiple Personality Disorders	

Discussion groups

alt.med.outpat.clinic, clari.tw.health, sci.med

Two Usenet newsgroups—sci.med and alt.med.outpat.clinic—will interest anyone looking for information on a specific disease or condition. Sci.med is also a Fidonet echo (Grand_Rounds), which is good news because many Fidonet users contribute useful information. If you can't find a medical newsgroup that matches your interests or needs, try following sci.med for a while. If you still don't see any relevant postings, ask for suggestions. Sci.med focuses on issues of interest to clinical health professionals, ranging from health ethics to medical office software. The alt.med.outpat.clinic newsgroup is a good place for patients to post specific health-related queries and get answers, including some from the Phriendly Physician, Dr. Burke Brian.

Doc in the Box
314-893-6099

Like Black Bag BBS, Doc in the Box offers a solid medical database and conference center that you can dial directly. Managed by Dr. Mark D. Winton, Doc in the Box gives you access to scores of medical discussion groups or conferences (from eight sources, including ADAnet, Fidonet, HealthCare Net, uucp newsgroups, and Safenet); hundreds of files; and about a dozen medical newsletters. Conference areas include such topics as psychobiology, AIDS, telemedicine, general medicine, nursing, chronic fatigue syndrome, diabetes, pharmacy, dentistry, immunology, nutrition, occupational medicine, medical physics, radiology, and medical transcription. Dr. Winton is active online and answers many questions posted by conference and newsgroup members. On the Internet, you'll also find him on several Usenet newsgroups.

Doc in the Box CBIS
(computer-based information service)

I first became interested in BBSs in 1986. I thought it was fascinating that you could call by modem to locate and retrieve files and information from far away. After calling around for a while, I saw an area that wasn't covered, namely, a medical-interest BBS. Since I enjoyed BBSing, I thought (like so many other sysops) that I would run my own BBS.

In 1988, I started Doc in the Box. It seemed a great way to provide up-to-date medical information. I set up a Wildcat Test Drive package with a 2400-baud modem and was amazed to see callers on a regular basis.

Over the years, the BBS has grown into a two-line system with software connecting to the Internet and Fidonet systems. I joined many networks and even ran a few.

The BBS allows me to post the *MMWR (Morbidity and Mortality Weekly Report)*, the National Institutes of Health (NIH) AIDS trials, and other medical journals and information, including a network for Americans with disabilities.

Many callers need anonymous information, so that's available. A number of my patients can keep up on medical developments as they happen. The BBS helps in my practice by keeping me on top of new information.

I have had a lot of good comments that this type of BBS provides files and messages not seen on any other. The key is networking with other systems. Almost no systems are islands anymore. Each is interconnected. The Internet, in turn, provides a massive group of BBSs that are connected.

I invite anyone to call Doc in the Box to see if there's any medical information that might be of interest to you or to a friend.

Mark_D Winton, M.D.

Duke University Medical Center
http://h-devil.www.mc.duke.edu/h-devil/

The Duke University Medical Center Home Page provides the usual information about various academic departments and branches of medicine. It also offers Healthy Devil Online, which addresses topics in emotional health, men's and women's health, nutrition, drinking and smoking, sexual health, and general health. You can submit your own question or read answers to hundreds of others posted online (listed by date and subject for each major category).

Duke University's Healthy Devil makes looking for answers to health questions fun.

Fam-Med Gopher

gopher://ftp.gac.edu/11/pub/E-mail-archives/fam-med

This gopher offers a smorgasbord of information related to family medicine. The Fam-Med gopher focuses on the use of computer and telecommunication technologies in both teaching and practicing family medicine. You can reach the conferences and files on this gopher from almost anywhere online—via e-mail, the Internet, Fidonet, CompuServe, and America Online. Everyone is invited to participate. You'll find archives of medically related newsletters and newsgroups, links to health-related gophers, electronic newsletters, medical shareware, and software reviews. The gopher is located in Minnesota at Gustavus Adolphus College (go into the Libraries and Reference directory, then into Medical References to get to Fam-Med).

Food and Drug Administration BBS

800-222-0185, 301-594-6849

The Food and Drug Administration (FDA) BBS offers free access to documents on nutrition labeling, consumer drug and medical device issues, and new drug approvals. You'll also find news releases, the Enforcement Report (weekly recall list), the Drug and Device Product Approvals List, medical devices and radiological health news, the FDA Medical Bulletin/MedWatch, AIDS treatment information, the FDA Consumer magazine (index and selected articles), FDA Federal Register summaries (available by subject or date), congressional testimony and speeches by FDA officials, upcoming FDA meetings, and import alerts. The BBS has an online user guide (also available in some local medical BBS file directories) and useful searching capabilities.

Health and Medicine in the News
gopher://lenti.med.umn.edu:71/11/news

This news-clipping service helps both the public and healthcare professionals keep up with the latest medical advances reported in medical literature and in the news media. Health and Medicine in the News cites newspaper articles published in Minnesota that report new medical research. You'll see this site listed in many medical school gophers and throughout the Internet. The service also offers a searchable gopher index that allows you to type in keywords to find articles of interest. You can also review a list of articles by date and topic. Accompanying most news article summaries is a citation of the medical journal article that sparked the news story.

– 67 –

The information superhighway offers a unique vehicle for obtaining medical information. By using one resource, Usenet newsgroups, people can ask questions about any illness. Often doctors, aware of the importance of communicating online medical information, respond to these questions.

Despite the altruism of some physicians, it's difficult to find doctors willing to offer services for the benefit and education of patients without expecting something in return. While participating in some newsgroups, like sci.med and sci.med.dentistry, I recognized the need for another source of medical information. Because of this, we created Health Watch Newsletter.

Our publication is published bimonthly. It has two main sections, medical and dental. With the help of Jose Garcia, M.D. and Ana V. Aviles, D.D.S., we provide information about almost any illness to our subscribers.

Through e-mail, subscribers have the opportunity to ask any question, which is forwarded to our contributing doctors for an answer. We then send answers back via e-mail to our subscribers and publish the information in Health Watch Newsletter for the benefit of all. We also accept contributions by organizations like the National Reye's Foundation and the Sjögren's Syndrome Foundation.

Our mailing list covers the United States and Europe. Health Watch Newsletter is free and supported only with donations. Anyone who wants to subscribe to the list can contact us at Hercilia@voyager.cris.com.

Janet M. Garcia, editor
Health Watch Newsletter

Health-Info

gopher://riceinfo.rice.edu/11/Safety/HealthInfo

Rice University offers several online clinics that provide information on health topics of particular interest to young adults. Directories include Women's Health (including information on contraception and breast cancer), Preventive Medicine (topics like diet, smoking, skin cancer, and heart disease), Food and Health, HIV/AIDS, Sexually Transmitted Diseases, Sports Medicine (including files on specific injuries and stretching), Texas Critters That Bite (like vicious squirrels), Illness (common disorders and eye problems), and Travel. While the site has a Texas flavor, you'll find much of the information helpful no matter where you live.

Health Info-Com
Network Medical Newsletter
mednews@asuvm.inre.asu.edu, bit.listserv.mednews

The Health Info-Com Network Medical Newsletter is a news digest edited by David Dodell, D.M.D. Subscribing to this newsletter will keep you abreast of key advances in medical research and clinical practice. A permanent address for the WWW version should also be available by now. An impressive staff of associate editors reviews the fully referenced articles. Occasionally, editorial notes accompany and complement specific articles. The newsletter also announces new online medical resources.

If you have time to read only one electronic medical newsletter, choose the Health Info-Com Newsletter. Remember, though, that Dr. Dodell writes this medical newsletter in his "spare" time. Take a moment to thank him for his services, and be patient if your subscription seems erratic at times.

Health Information
gopher://vixen.cso.uiuc.edu: 70/11/UI/CSF/health/heainfo

Of the university-based health information servers, the University of Illinois' gopher is probably the most useful. You'll find a wide array of comprehensive health information in well-stocked directories such as Diseases/Conditions, Drug/Alcohol, Health Promotion, Fitness, Nutrition, Sexuality, Stress, Tests, Translated Materials, Women's Health, and Medications. The information is current and thorough. The gopher also carries the *Mortality and Morbidity Weekly Report* (*MMWR*) from the Centers for Disease Control and Prevention in Atlanta.

Healthline
gopher://healthline.umt.edu:700/

The University of Montana's Student Health Services provide Healthline, an online service that offers the same type of information you'd receive at most university health centers. Menus in Healthline contain documents on several topics including sexuality, drug and alcohol information, and about 50 common disorders such as migraine headaches, depression, and irritable bowel syndrome. Healthline also contains links to other gopher servers. A real advantage of Healthline is that it provides a wide range of easily accessible, general health-related information. Be sure to read Tips on Using Healthline in the General Information directory before using the service.

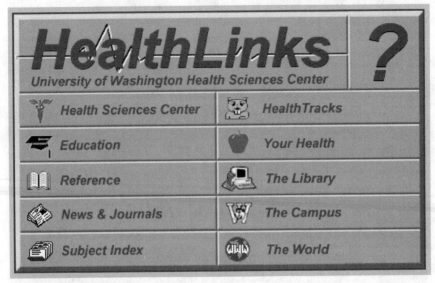

HealthLinks is a great place to find health information and perform medical searches.

HealthLinks

http://www.hslib.washington.edu/

The University of Washington's HealthLinks provides useful consumer health information, excellent searching capabilities, and, as the name implies, links to other online medical resources. The Web page is well-organized and easy to use for researching medical topics, and provides access to news clipping and reference services not normally provided by a health information server.

The Your Health directory is full of timely, informative news articles written by the University of Washington Health Sciences news and community relations staff in collaboration with faculty. The HealthTracks gopher includes directories with links to resources on clinical care, biomedical sciences, community and public health, healthcare reform, medical informatics and technology, and other health gophers.

Among its wealth of additional resources, HealthLinks provides access to Web-searching tools such as WebCrawler, Yahoo, Lycos, and WWW Worm, as well as Web sites that offer hierarchically arranged medical information and resources (such as Health & Bioscience Guides, Medical Matrix, CERN Web Guide, EINet Galaxy, and Yahoo Guide).

Health Online
310-831-6775

If you don't have Internet access or an account with an online service (and even if you do), you shouldn't miss Health Online, a BBS devoted to health and healthcare issues that makes it easy for even the novice computer user to download files, leave messages, and chat with other users.

Conference areas and files are available for both healthcare professionals and people interested in their own health. You'll find information on both tradition-al and alternative therapies. Also available is a session with Eliza, the Computer Psychologist, who concludes each session with: "Thanks for coming to me for therapy. The fee for this session is $75.00. Please press a key once you've written out your check payable to Eliza." Health Online also offers com-puter support at the Computer Help Desk. For users afraid of computer viruses, you'll be relieved to know Health Online examines all files for viruses prior to posting for access and download.

Health Services

gopher://genesis.ait.psu.edu/ 11/psuinfo/Health%20Services

Penn State University's Health Services gopher provides information on cancer, drugs, alcohol, smoking, eyes, skin, nutrition, sexual concerns, women's health, and other general health issues. The information on nutrition is extensive, with helpful reports on vitamins, organic foods, vegetarianism, sports nutrition, and nutrition during pregnancy. However, the service targets primarily young adults, with few files addressing health concerns in children or older adults.

The universality of medicine makes it unique among professions. Not all of us will need lawyers in our lifetimes. Some of us will stubbornly continue to prepare our own taxes. But each of us will eventually require the services of a physician. In certain countries, such services might often be beyond our financial means. So where does that leave us? It leaves us in the dark with respect to one of the most essential components of human happiness—our health.

In my view, online medicine attempts to reduce the inequities inherent within our capitalist social system. Through online medicine, anyone with either a computer or valid library card has access to medical knowledge—and hence power. Individuals who once felt completely shut out by the seemingly magical powers of modern medicine are now included more than ever. People are less helpless when they have access to information. They are free at last.

Of course, online medicine is no replacement for personal patient care. Rather, it functions as a crucial supplement to it. Through online advice, patients have the beauty of choice. Is further testing merited? Do I need to see a doctor now? Next month? Or is the problem one that will be resolved on its own and need not concern me at all?

For me, the chief incentive for offering online medical help is the monumental amount of anxiety I can alleviate with a few taps on my friendly keyboard. Often it is therapeutic for patients simply to know someone is out there listening. On the Internet, no one rushes you out of the doctor's office. And while some people might consider computer contact an impersonal version of the real thing, it's not quite so. Many individuals are able to open up and bare their souls online in a way they're not able to in person.

Far from depersonalizing the doctor-patient relationship, online medicine reshapes it, providing more balance and poise without the ulterior motives. Online I stand to make no money from the amount of tests the patient undergoes and to lose no money from the amount of time the patient spends in my "office."

Online medicine offers a beneficial service to all of humanity's diverse members. People can receive knowledge, advice, and, at times, friendship. They can converse on level ground with physicians in the unhurried and laid-back universe of the Internet. Paradoxically, while propelling us full-steam ahead into the future, online medicine takes us back to our roots when healthcare's primary focus was people and sharing rather than lab tests, money, and power.

Brian A. Burke, M.D.

HealthSource BBS
813-979-7307

If you have health-related questions, HealthSource BBS has Answers, a place where anyone dialing in with a modem can post questions (anonymously, if desired) to be answered by a physician. You can also read hundreds of previous questions and answers. HealthSource BBS, supported by University Community Hospital in Tampa, Fla. and operated by Jay Reese, M.D. (with help from other physicians), is available free of charge 24 hours a day, 7 days a week. You'll see responses to questions about diet, fitness, specific symptoms, specific diseases, medication use and side effects, dental and eye problems, parenting issues, and sexual health. While HealthSource provides answers to your questions, it won't provide the dozens of network conferences and newsgroup echoes that many other medical BBSs offer. As with all online medical resources, HealthSource is an educational service only and should not replace advice from your doctor.

Healthwise

http://www.cc.columbia.edu:80/cu/healthwise/

Healthwise, the Health Education and Wellness program of the Columbia University Health Service, is another site that offers answers to your health questions. You'll want to read the Health Service's online newsletter and visit Go Ask Alice!, an interactive question-and-answer health line covering Sexual Health and Relationships, Drugs and Alcohol, Nutrition and Healthy Diet, Emotional Well-Being, and General Health. Although hundreds of archived answers already exist, Alice answers about a dozen new questions anonymously and publicly each week. Alice is blunt in her answers but also thorough, often providing the latest medical research. If you want a confidential answer, Alice can send it directly to your e-mail address, but the response can take up to two weeks since this service is very popular.

Healthwise is the Health Education and Wellness program of Columbia University Health Service. We are a team of professional and peer educators committed to helping you make choices that will contribute to your personal health and happiness, the well-being of others, and to the planet we share.

The star of Columbia University's Healthwise service is Alice, who answers your questions.

Journal Watch

jwatch@world.std.com

Bimonthly on the Usenet sci.med newsgroup, you'll see the table of contents and the two top stories from Journal Watch, a medical literature survey produced by the Massachusetts Medical Society. You can subscribe to the full newsletter electronically or via U.S. mail. Journal Watch's physician editors compile summaries of the leading clinical research stories from major journals, such as *The Journal of the American Medical Association*, *New England Journal of Medicine*, *Science*, *The Lancet*, *Annals of Internal Medicine*, *Archives of Internal Medicine*, and many more. The free posting to sci.med offers an easy way to stay abreast of the latest and most important clinical findings in the medical literature.

Med Help International

516-423-0472, http://medhlp.netusa.net/

Med Help International is another general medical information BBS worth reviewing. An international team of physicians and healthcare professionals volunteer their time and expertise to provide medical information in simple language to patients and their families. Information also comes from research institutes, universities, government agencies, medical support groups, and public and private medical groups. You can browse through Med Help's extensive medical library or go to the public forums to meet other people who have similar medical problems. All information is free. You can use Med Help's customized research services to request information on specific medical topics, for which Med Help requests a $20 donation. You can also access the BBS information through Med Help's Web site, telnet connection, or FTP site. At the Web site, you'll find many links to other online health and medical resources.

National Institutes of Health (NIH)

http://www.nih.gov

This site is of primary interest to researchers and healthcare professionals who want information on grant and contract announcements, molecular biology and molecular modeling, and research opportunities. It also provides an NIH calendar of events, among other items. You'll find links to individual institutes and other medical resources, which offer information for patients. As more NIH offices come online, check here to locate them.

National Institutes of Health Information Center
800-644-2271, 301-480-5144

You can't beat the NIH Information Center's 800 number for downloading medical documents and images. This BBS serves students, medical professionals, reporters, science writers, and the public with information about the NIH and medical research it supports. When you sign on to the NIH Information Center, the system immediately lists 800 numbers for voice information on several health topics, including AIDS, cancer, and Alzheimer's disease.

The Information Center offers the following: an NIH Information Index (list of diseases under investigation at the NIH and persons to contact), NIH publications, press releases, healthline news and features (articles from the scientific literature translated into language the public can understand), calendars, images, an NIH almanac, NIH history, clinical alerts, computer utilities, general health information publications (full text), articles prepared by NIH that appeared in *The Journal of the American Medical Association*, as well as information on an environmental task force and alternative medicine. In addition, this BBS contains bulletins on selected topics, including descriptions of other online information sources and toll-free help lines.

New York State Department of Health
gopher://gopher.health.state.ny.us/1

On this gopher, you'll find general health-related information and convenient access to data resources. Since this service is provided for New York residents, you'll also find local information about New York facility locations, health information services, and state and county health statistics. The Consumer Health Information directory offers a collection of reading materials on a variety of medical subjects. You can search the directories or the index itself for documents on cancer, communicable diseases, environmental and occupational health, heart disease, and women's health. Topics of general interest with New York-specific information include home care, nursing homes, hospitals, community services, and vital records.

University Health Service
gopher://gopher.uhs.uga.edu:70/1

This keyword-searchable gopher server offers the usual array of health information, primarily of interest to young adults. You'll find directories full of documents on general health (including allergic rhinitis, warts, bacterial meningitis, and ingrown toenails), sexual health (including a good overview of men's health), mental health, and women's health. The service's HealthCall newsletters are also online and include a number of general interest articles. If you don't find the information you want here, you can use convenient links to health information servers at the University of Montana, Pennsylvania State University, the University of Illinois, Wake Forest University, and the University of Wisconsin.

University of Wisconsin
gopher://gopher.adp.wisc.edu:70/
11/.browse/.METACACDI/.CACDI05

The information files available at the University of Wisconsin gopher server might appeal to a wider audience than files at most other academic health centers. The main directories cover Alcohol and Other Drugs, Bites and Parasitic Infections, Cancer, Contraception, Emotional Health, Environmental Health, Fitness, Food and Health, Internal Affairs (including high blood pressure, viral hepatitis, epilepsy, and toxic shock syndrome), It's All in Your Head, Muscles, Bones and Joints, Sexual Health, and Skin and Tissues. Check this site if you can't find a short blurb on a common condition elsewhere on the Internet.

Virtual Hospital
http://indy.radiology.uiowa.edu/VirtualHospital.html

The University of Iowa's Virtual Hospital provides a continuously updated medical multimedia database for use in physician education and support of patient care. You'll find online, multimedia textbooks that feature audio, video, and high-resolution images. This site isn't particularly useful for patients seeking medical information, although the Iowa Health Book is an excellent resource. You'll also find The Virtual Children's Hospital, which offers information for pediatricians and others providing care to children, and links to many other online medical resources.

World Health Organization
gopher.who.ch, http://www.who.ch/

The World Health Organization (WHO) offers both gopher and Web servers that provide information about the WHO and its major programs, as well as press releases, newsletters, updates on international travel and health (such as advice, vaccination requirements, and warnings), Usenet news, and FAQs. You'll also find links to other health-related servers and several search engines and indexing tools. Because the WHO server is in Switzerland, you might get stalled in traffic when trying to connect. However, if you're looking for answers to your international health questions, it's worth the trip.

Commercial services
America Online

keyword CONSUMER REPORTS Although *Consumer Reports* evaluates mainly cars, finances, electronic equipment, and other household items, you'll still be able to search for medical features and read the complete article. (For convenience, *Consumer Reports* divides the articles into separate files so you don't have to scroll through one large document to find what you want.) The Home Workshop menu includes health-related articles, including buying vitamins, carbon monoxide detectors, and coffee and health.

keyword HEALTH The Better Health and Medical Forum offers an informed, supportive online community with hundreds of articles by professional health writers. You'll find medical issues grouped in the following categories: Multimedia Self-Care Showcase, Lifestyles and Wellness, Mental Health and Addictions, Human Sexuality, Informed Decisions, Health Reform and Insurance, Men/Women/Children's Health, Senior's Health and Caregiving, Alternative Medicine, and Home Medical Guide. You can search, by keyword, from anywhere in the forum. The Forum provides links to disABILITIES and other health resources on AOL. You'll find software, documents, images, quizzes, and many more downloadable files for all topics discussed. You'll also be able to join scheduled conferences, informal gatherings, and support groups in the Health and Medical chat area. The message center encourages discussion among patients, caregivers, healthcare professionals, and other interested people.

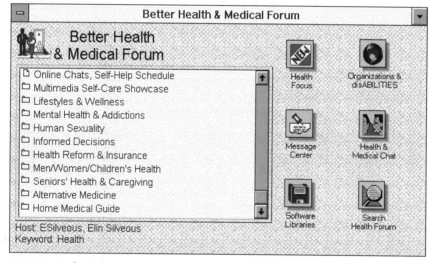

America Online's Better Health & Medical Forum covers a wide range of health topics.

keyword HEALTHFOCUS HealthFocus provides detailed coverage of health headlines through opinion polls, interviews with online members, articles, photographs, artwork, computer graphics, discussions, and debates. The central theme of HealthFocus changes regularly, and former topics are archived. Lively debates cover controversial aspects of the main topic. You'll find glossaries, clinical alerts, research highlights, signs and symptoms, trivia and fact sheets, preventive measures, treatment options, multimedia documents, downloadable files, and news headlines all devoted to one medical issue, such as Alzheimer's or heart disease. Check HealthFocus to see if the Forum is covering or has covered a concern of yours. If so, you can make a one-stop information shopping trip.

keyword NAS The National Academy of Sciences, home to the Institute of Medicine, has many online documents addressing fluoridated water, vaccinations, the abortion pill RU-486, genetic testing, the Women's Health Initiative, lead exposure risks, fetal research, cancer risk assessment, AIDS research, and a wide range of other cutting-edge medical topics. You can use a keyword search.

CompuServe

go APO2 Associated Press Online offers science and health articles, as well as other headline options.

go CNN The CNN Forum offers an interactive version of this 24-hour news network. You can check the Health message board to discuss and debate CNN medical stories. You can search the Forum's libraries for transcripts of many stories, along with contact numbers, resources, and photographs. In the CNN Conference rooms, you can join online interviews with international experts and CNN staffers.

go COLUMNS Among the syndicated columns available through CompuServe, you'll find one devoted to women's health (Her Health, by Leslie Laurence) and one to men's health (His Health, by Dr. Ken Goldberg). You can also read The Medical Adviser (a question-and-answer column), produced by the Palo Alto Medical Foundation with a database that contains articles from more than 3,500 medical journals around the world.

go ENS ($$) CompuServe's Executive News Service can keep you informed of health and medical news. ENS is an electronic news-clipping service that monitors several news wires for stories containing keywords you specify. These stories are "clipped" and stored in folders for you to review.

go GOODHEALTH ($) The Health and Fitness Forum covers a broad range of issues, from drug and alcohol addiction to women's health, from chronic fatigue syndrome to self-help. Members discuss wellness-related matters, including nutrition, mental health, child care, aging, and fitness. There are specific sections for swimming, running, body building, and martial arts. Many healthcare professionals (physicians, educators, pharmacists, counselors, physiologists, nurses, therapists, and others) participate in the forum, including Dr. Michael Mayer, who presides over the Doctor's Inn. Several 12-step real-time meetings are held every week, with the focus, time, and location for each posted online. Forum libraries correspond to individual message sections.

go HEALTH This directory points you to consumer-oriented medical resources offered by CompuServe, including HealthNet, Consumer Reports Complete Drug Reference, the Handicapped User's Database, health support forums, Healthy Living (also accessible directly via GO HLT-4), AIDS information, NORD services, syndicated columns on health topics, Health Database Plus, and PaperChase (MEDLINE). Healthy Living provides additional pointers to the Health & Fitness Forum, the Holistic Health Forum, Human Sexuality, Information USA, the Retirement Living Forum, and the Time Warner Lifestyles Forum.

go HNT CompuServe's HealthNet Reference Library is probably the best single source of general health and medical information offered by any commercial service. You'll find answers to most health-related questions you have. You can look for information according to individual disease, disorder, symptom, medication, first aid procedure, surgical procedure, test, medical procedure, eye-care concern, reproductive health concern, or obstetrics topic. HealthNet articles are written by physicians and other healthcare professionals who are experts in their respective fields.

go MEDICAL This directory points you to every major medical and health-related resource offered by CompuServe. Included are links to the AMIA Forum, the Cancer Forum, the Diabetes Forum, the Health & Fitness Forum, the Comprehensive Core Medical Library, HealthNet, NORD services, Physician Data Query, PsycINFO, Health Database Plus, Business Database Plus, IQuest Medical InfoCenter, PaperChase (MEDLINE), and the UK Professionals Forum.

go MEDSIG ($) The American Medical Informatics Association (AMIA) Forum assists in the exchange of medical information and the use of computers in medically related activities. Although the AMIA forum provides a section to ask healthcare questions, the forum exists primarily to promote discussion about medical applications of computers. The libraries contain medical shareware and other resources related to the use of computers in medicine. The message sections address several issues of concern to health professionals, such as office systems, health policy and legal issues, research and bioethics, and medical records. The Forum offers message sections for family practitioners, pediatricians, obstetricians, gynecologists, nonprimary-care specialists, critical care, emergency medicine, dentists, mental health professionals, and pathologists. Other healthcare professionals are encouraged to join as well.

Delphi

go CUSTOM 014 The Consumer Medicine and Public Health SIG keeps you abreast of current events in medicine. Topics include diabetes, cancer, pain, death and dying, chronic disease, computers in medicine, and more. Host Robert S. Pataki, M.D. encourages members to be involved, and updates the large database regularly. You'll find the forum a lively place for exchanging information and sharing personal experiences.

go CUSTOM 147 Living Healthy—the Spa at Delphi is a virtual health spa where you can discuss any concerns about your mental or physical health. The group covers the full spectrum of mind/body wellness, with topics including mental health, autism, developmental disorders, recovery from addictions, massage, exercise, health, beauty, and physical illnesses. You can also join several health-related newsgroups.

e•World

shortcut LIVING WELL Living Well brings you Culinary Cues, Health & Fitness (an "owner's manual for your body"), and Assignment: Earth. The Health & Fitness section provides links to The Family Doctor, Energy Express, and The Health Club (message center). Dr. Allan Bruckheim (The Family Doctor) writes a column about common health concerns, sometimes posting answers to questions posed by online readers (although he doesn't respond personally). The Family

Doctor has covered items such as Rogaine, vaginitis, chronic fatigue syndrome, carpal tunnel syndrome, infertility, aging, Parkinson's disease, skin care, breast implants, ulcer treatment, and many other specific medical problems.

shortcut TRANSFORMATIONS Transformations covers 12-step groups, medical issues, and mental health concerns. If you're interested in self-help, Transformations can lead you to online workshops, classes, and support group meetings. Turn to Beginning the Journey for self-help resources, national help lines, and health information. You'll find longer files in the Idea Exchange. You'll find text information and self-help support for attention deficit disorder; Alzheimer's; cancer; chronic fatigue syndrome; heart disease; HIV/AIDS; sexually transmitted diseases; lupus; and Paget's, Parkinson's, and Raynaud's diseases, among others. There's also information available on aging, death and dying, respiratory problems, medications, and women's health.

shortcut UPI UPI News You Can Use offers health and medicine news from around the world. Articles are updated as late-breaking developments occur.

shortcut USA TODAY Through USA Today Decisionlines (select Industries), you'll have access to headlines and abstracts about top health stories in the United States. You can find stories up to five days old in the Decisionlines archives.

– 83 –

GEnie

keyword MEDICAL In GEnie's Medical RoundTable, you can go to Category 2 to look for answers to common medical questions and information about health issues. In Category 6, you can pose questions to a physician. You can also find general health information about specific diseases and conditions in Category 5, which includes dozens of support groups. In addition, there's the Health News & Issues newsletter, which reports on major news in the medical field.

keyword QUIKNEWS ($$) For regular updates on a particular medical topic, GEnie QuikNews allows you to select terms for full-text searches of incoming stories from Reuters World Service. If the headline or body of a story matches one of your search terms, the story will be sent to you via GE Mail.

Prodigy

jump AP ONLINE AP Online offers the latest national and international health and science news. For background material on current top health stories, jump BACKGROUND, which provides links to Prodigy's online encyclopedia.

jump CONSUMER REPORTS You can also find *Consumer Reports* articles online on Prodigy. Health & Fitness topics include drugs and medicine, infection and diseases, health products, medical treatments, injury and medical emergency, insurance, genetics, organ systems, lifestyle, and other broad categories of articles. Among the Foods & Beverages topics are articles on food safety, nutrition labels, diet and nutrition, and the individual food groups. After you select an article, you've given a one-sentence introduction to the topic. You then can proceed to individual sections (described by subhead titles) of your choice. You can also read A Question of Health, a question-and-answer column about medical treatments and health products.

jump HEALTH BB ($) Health BB covers a broad number and scope of topics, so keep digging through subdirectories until you find what you're looking for. If you don't see what you want in the main topic list, check the Other topic. The first screen (one of many) includes subjects like About ADD, About Marijuana, About Smoking, AIDS, Air Cleaners, Aloe Vera, and Alternative Medicine, typical for the range of conversations taking place here. Another good place to check is Family Medicine. Fortunately, you can search the subject lists by keyword to track down the threads you want to read.

jump HEALTH/FITNESS The Health/Fitness directory provides you with links to Health News, Health Topics, Consumer Reports, Keeping Fit, Health BB, and health and fitness-related advertisements.

jump HEALTH NEWS ($) Health News offers five leading medical headlines, a weekly roundup of the 20 top health news stories, and links to online Consumer Reports, the Health BB, Health Topics, and Keeping Fit, as well as general science news.

jump HEALTH TOPICS Jump to Health Topics for the following six health options: Diseases (Alzheimer's disease, AIDS, allergies, cancer, strokes, women's health, and headaches, among others); Children; Wellness; Brain and Behavior; Exercise and Sports; and Hot Topics. After you select an individual article, you'll read either a wire or news story or a Health Topics document.

jump MEDICAL SUPPORT BB ($) The Medical Support BB provides a forum where Prodigy members with medical concerns can support one another. You can attend conferences in the Medical Auditorium or join many smaller groups to talk about specific diseases or disorders in the Medical Support chat area. You'll find Ask A Specialist in the Other Medical topic. Healthcare specialists who help include cardiologists, chiropractors, dentists, dermatologists, podiatrists, urologists, allergists, optometrists, obstetrician/gynecologists, orthopedists, plastic surgeons, neurologists, endocrinologists, child therapists, physical therapists, midwives, and pharmacists. The Other Medical topic covers many health issues, including breast implant concerns, Lyme disease, pregnancy and birth announcements, and a subject called Julia Tupler, which includes information about this nurse's Maternal Fitness Program.

6
AIDS and HIV infection

*I*f you're looking for information about AIDS or HIV infection, you won't be disappointed. Online you'll find extensive AIDS databases and wide-ranging support groups. You can download everything from grim statistics to AIDS art to reports of work in developing an AIDS vaccine by the late Dr. Jonas Salk. The Centers for Disease Control and Prevention's National AIDS Clearinghouse provides information on more than 11,000 educational materials and 18,000 organizations that offer HIV- and AIDS-related services. You can find excellent resources on gopher servers, Web pages, BBSs, and commercial online services. Anyone with a computer and a modem can access a well-established network of dedicated individuals and organizations committed both to advancing scientific progress in preventing and treating AIDS and to ensuring quality, compassionate care for those with the disease or HIV infection.

The resources included in this chapter will point you to hundreds of other online (and offline) AIDS resources not described here. Several academic institutions maintain well-stocked AIDS directories, including Yale and Johns Hopkins (see chapter 15, Searching for medical resources), the University of California (San Francisco, Santa Cruz, Davis), and the University of Southern California. Gopher servers and Web pages at these sites will give you access to the major online AIDS resources and documents. At many sites, you'll also find electronic newsletters and BBSs we haven't described here because of the rapidly growing number of them available.

AIDS Education General Information System (AEGIS)
714-248-2836

If you use your modem to get AIDS information, you need to sign on to AEGIS. Established in 1990 by the Sisters of St. Elizabeth of Hungary, AEGIS has established itself as the leading AIDS information resource in the United States and as the cornerstone of the Global Electronic Network for AIDS (GENA), an international consortium of BBSs. Here you'll find the latest AIDS news, browse medical journals and newsletter articles, exchange information with friends or colleagues, and join lively debates.

Most information is in two areas, Conferences and the AIDS Online Database & File Library. The library features one of the world's largest nongovernmental, electronic file libraries devoted to AIDS. There are more than 160,000 records from AmFAR (American Foundation for AIDS Research), the Centers for Disease Control and Prevention, the U.S. Public Health Service, and a host of international AIDS organizations. The library is divided into 10 databases searchable by keywords and a download area. The Conferences section has four network areas—AEGIS, Fidonet, HIVNET, and the Internet. The Conferences and message areas pass electronic mail between individual BBSs in the AEGIS Network and Fidonet. Users who support the service financially can use a QWK offline reader and Internet e-mail. The AEGIS network has member BBSs in 22 states and Canada. With more BBSs always joining, you might find one that provides you local access.

– 87 –

AIDS Info BBS
415-626-1246, gopher://itsa.ucsf.edu:70/11/.i/.q/.d

As the name indicates, Ben Gardiner's AIDS Info BBS is a comprehensive bulletin board that serves the education and support needs of HIV-positive individuals, people with AIDS, and others concerned about AIDS. Access has been free since July 25, 1985. You can reach this BBS by either dialing up with your modem or going to its mirror location at the University of California, San Francisco gopher. Many other AIDS-related gopher servers and Web pages pro-

```
 1> Articles            :  [4704 items] News, Articles, Book Reviews
 2> Q & A               :  Commonly Asked Questions
 3> OPEN FORUM          :  [6743+ items] Public message area
 4> Resources           :  Names & phone lists
 5> Library Files       :  Statistics, Stored Daily Summaries
 6> Daily news items    :  summarized from publications everywhere
 7> Therapies           :  Discussions, Threads, & Reports
 8> Periodicals         :   [516 items]  Newsletters
 9> Calender            :  Scheduled events on AIDS
10> About this System   :  Information, Help and History
11> Utilities           :  Change User Settings
12> What, Index, Who    :  What's new, who called; word research
21> KEYWORD(s) SEARCH   :  one or two words
22> ITEM COUNT          :  prints the actual count
23> PROTOCOL DOWNLOAD   :  via XMODEM
 h> Help.
 e> E-Mail.
 d> Directory of topics.
 g> Goodbye. Terminate session.

Top Level: Enter selection (or ?):
```

The AIDS Info BBS offers thousands of files to read online or download.

vide a link to the BBS. When using the system, you can create an alias user name. The interface is easy to follow and offers help. In both the BBS and gopher mirror, you can use keywords or an index to search the directories. You can search through more than 12,000 documents, including articles, FAQs, statistics, library files, daily news items, therapy discussions and reports, newsletters, and scheduled events on AIDS. You can also join the open forum for public discussions of AIDS-related topics.

Centers for Disease Control and Prevention (CDC) National AIDS Clearinghouse (NAC)

gopher://cdcnac.aspensys.com:72
(http:// and ftp:// also work with this address)

You'll find a directory for the CDC NAC included in many gopher servers, Web pages, and BBSs, or you can go there directly. Besides the CDC NAC gopher site, the government also operates CDC NAC Online, which is free for researchers and healthcare professionals, but isn't accessible to the public. Users of CDC NAC Online must obtain a password to access the tremendous databases available. At the public gopher site, you'll find the latest news and announcements about many crucial AIDS- and HIV-related issues, including prevention and education campaigns, treatment and clinical trials, legislation and regulation, and upcoming events. The *Morbidity and Mortality Weekly Report* (*MMWR*) is available here as well. The CDC Clearinghouse also disseminates information via the sci.med.aids newsgroup on the Internet.

Conversational hypertext access technology (CHAT)
telnet debra.dgbt.doc.ca 3000

Do you want to enjoy a new technology while learning about AIDS? Try making a telnet connection to CHAT, an information retrieval technology developed by Drs. Thomas Whalen and Andrew Patrick at Industry Canada. CHAT is based on a hypertext model (like the World Wide Web) in which paragraphs of information link together. Unlike other hypertext systems, however, CHAT uses software to perform the navigation transparently so you see only the natural language dialog. In other words, you ask questions in normal English sentences and CHAT answers. If you feel shy about asking a computer questions, you can browse the system by hitting Return for more specific information or ?–Return (both keys together) for more general information. CHAT is surprisingly fast and responsive. While it isn't necessarily the place to do serious research, you'll find it faster and easier to ask basic questions here than perform keyword searches anywhere else, not to mention you'll have fun doing it.

Discussion groups

People seeking support and information about HIV infection and AIDS can find dozens of mailing lists and newsgroups, only a very small portion of which are listed here:

AIDS: aids-request@cs.ucla.edu
AIDS: listserv@rutgers.edu

```
Type a Question or Press ENTER to browse:
Do more men than women have AIDS?

The Computer Says:
In July 1987, it was reported that equal proportions of male and
female military applicants from San Francisco and New York were
infected with the AIDS virus. In Africa, where AIDS has been
spreading since the 1950's, equal numbers of men and women have
AIDS. Clearly AIDS is not limited to  male homosexuals. Anyone who
engages in high-risk activities is in danger of becoming infected
with the AIDS virus.

Type a Question or Press ENTER to browse:

Tell me more. . .

The Computer Says:

A person who does not engage in high-risk activities and who has a
single sexual partner who does not engage in high-risk activities
has a very low risk of becoming infected with AIDS. Some people are
concerned that they may get infected with the AIDS virus through a
blood transfusion. Since antibody testing began in March 1985, there
is only about one chance in ten million that a blood transfusion
will cause an infection.

Type a Question or Press ENTER to browse:
```

You can telnet to Canada to chat about AIDS.

AIDS Stat: aids-stat-request@wubios.wustl.edu

HIV-AIDS-ARC: majordomo@hivnet.org

HIV-AIDS-Data: majordomo@hivnet.org

HIV-AIDS-Dialogue: majordomo@hivnet.org

HIV-AIDS-HIV: majordomo@hivnet.org

HIV-AIDS-Spiritual: majordomo@hivnet.org

HIV-AIDS-Women: majordomo@hivnet.org

bionet.molbio.hiv

clari.tw.health.aids

hiv.aids.issues

hiv.aidsweekly

hiv.alt-treatments

hiv.atn

hiv.med.questions

hiv.resources.addresses

hiv.women

misc.health.aids

sci.med.aids

Many of these groups are echoed on Fidonet, which also has several conferences of its own. You can subscribe to these discussion groups as you would any newsgroup or mailing list (you'll find the instructions in chapter 1, *The Internet*. To subscribe to mailing lists that start with -request@, just send an e-mail note asking to be placed on the list. Of these discussion groups, the oldest and most active is sci.med.aids, which covers a broad range of AIDS-related topics. This moderated group addresses the causes of AIDS and opportunistic infections, AIDS vaccines and drugs, and AIDS prevention and education. To avoid posting dangerous and undocumented therapies, newsgroup moderators require references for unconventional medical or research claims. Sci.med.aids also posts several publications, including CDC AIDS Daily Summary, AIDS Treatment News, and The Veterans Administration AIDS Info Newsletter.

The language of the heart via computer

I lost my husband of 25 years to AIDS, and swiftly on the wings of his flight two close friends followed. Numb from the feeling of despair, I stumbled through countless days trying to find some meaning and purpose to my existence. One doesn't simply make the transition from quasi-scientist, caregiver, advocate, masseuse, etc., to sedentary, sullen singlehood in a matter of days. I rode the treadmill of anger, rage, and self-pity until I came careening in for a crash landing. My fundamental problem was the isolation, admittedly by choice.

Over the next few months, I found myself in perpetual motion with my thoughts moving so rapidly I could barely keep up with them. I began initially by amusing myself with the wonderful world of computer communication, which fortunately I could do from home at my leisure. What began as a mere diversion escalated into a part-time job keeping pace with the amount of letters I received. This wasn't like sitting in a friend's living room over a cup of coffee or chatting on the phone. This was an ethereal connection, where one heart speaks to another.

There was a voluminous amount of medical advice, research data, treatment information (medical and holistic), forums for ethical debates, and more, right at my fingertips. This was an integral part of my achieving the status of "HIV/AIDS expert." Humbly, I might add. I became a human channel of information I could use in my volunteer work with our local AIDS Committee. My involvement has been primarily in public health education, and I travel when I can to share my message with different communities on family dynamics and psychosocial issues. Whether I'm speaking to a room of health professionals or a home for unwed teenage mothers, I usually manage to generate a lot of interest and feedback when I enlighten them about my relationship with people around the world. None of this would have been financially feasible without my steadfast union with the Internet.

It's difficult to fathom oneself talking to someone in Australia, Jerusalem, or the Yukon Territories for over an hour, without the stress of high overhead, undue delays, miscommunication problems, or physical burnout!! But it's the only effective means that I use to travel across the world within minutes to step inside of someone's life. The main attraction for computer addicts, albeit "terminal talkers" like myself, is the freedom of expression it affords the individual in sharing one-on-one at the gut level. Computers are less invasive, and at the very worst someone might drop you, like a bad cold. However, I have yet to encounter a single individual who wasn't willing to disclose their humanness.

Being merely mortal, I was becoming too stressed keeping up with the monumental needs that families struggling with HIV/AIDS have to cope with. That vital connection to another who can identify with how you feel is a life-sustaining support system in the haunting face of fear and crisis. Inspired by all those to whom I grew so attached, I initiated the creation of a newsgroup that deals solely and exclusively with psychosocial issues. It was my intention to establish a network that would link people with others in an atmosphere of compassion, open-mindedness, and acceptance.

This experience has been a powerful motivator for me. I continue to maintain close ties with people from all parts of the globe. It's my way of staying in touch with myself and the world that exists around me. In the information age, no one can argue that technology is a powerful source of empowerment, both in seeking knowledge and disseminating it. It's my way of receiving, processing, and transmitting my growing awareness of HIV/AIDS, and the crucial need to communicate through the language of the heart.

Anne M. Cameron

Global Electronic Network for Aids (GENA)

gopher gopher.hivnet.org,
FTP ftp.hivnet.org, http://www.hivnet.org

Based in Amsterdam, GENA is a worldwide network for HIV and AIDS information and discussion. GENA comprises HIVNET (a gopher and Web page based in Europe), AEGIS, the Association for Progressive Communications (via Greennet and Gaylink), and several other online organizations. You can reach GENA via Fidonet (through HIVNET or AEGIS nodes), gopher, WWW, and e-mail. Because this is an international server, the documents come in several languages— English, German, French, Dutch, and Russian.

The GENA server offers AIDS art, calendars of events associated with several organizations around the world, myriad lists of resources, dozens of electronic newsletters and periodicals, message boards, AIDS conference abstracts, and thousands of library files. In addition, HIVNET provides online treatment information from Project Inform, a leading U.S. AIDS treatment information and advocacy organization. Among Project Inform's treatment offerings are an Introductory Treatment Packet, several fact sheets, and two publications (Project Inform Perspective and Briefing Paper).

You can perform simple full-text searches of the AIDS Information Newsletter, AIDS Treatment News, BETA (Bulletin of Experimental Treatments for AIDS) Online, Being Alive, Body Positive Newsletter (U.K.), Body Positive Online

Magazine, CDC Aids Daily Summaries, Community Aids Treatment Exchange, Gay Men's Health Crisis Treatment Issues, and Health Info-Com Newsletter. You can also receive much of this information via e-mail and access the archives of all discussion groups and newsletters via gopher (GENA Mailing List Archives) and FTP (/gopher/newsgroups). If you're connecting via anonymous FTP, look for a file called Where_to_find_files that shows the links between gopher menu titles and the actual directories.

Global Programme on AIDS (GPA)
gopher://gopher.who.ch:70/11/.gpa/

Accessible by WWW (through WHO at http://www.who.ch/) and gopher, you'll find this World Health Organization site the best source of international research news about AIDS. GPA Docbase contains the full text of WHO publications on AIDS, including volumes in the WHO AIDS series. The site also provides meeting reports (Paris AIDS Summit, for example), pamphlets, public speeches, and other statements from the Global Programme on AIDS. Although GPA attempts to reproduce complete original documents, technical limitations at the gopher site prevent the inclusion of some charts, tables, illustrations, and other information. However, some of these might have been added to the Web pages. You'll also find access to most other online AIDS resources (FAQs, HIVNET, NIAID, sci.med.aids, and other resources) in addition to the GPA FTP server.

Kairos Support for Caregivers
http://www.catalog.com/kairos/welcome.htm

Kairos helps caregivers of HIV-infected people, take better care of themselves. Kairos is a nonprofit, community-service agency. You can download material from Kairos, learn about the organization itself, and find dozens of excellent links to other online AIDS and HIV resources, including the AIDS Virtual Library, AIDS BBS, the NAC, HIVNET, and AIDS Information Newsletter.

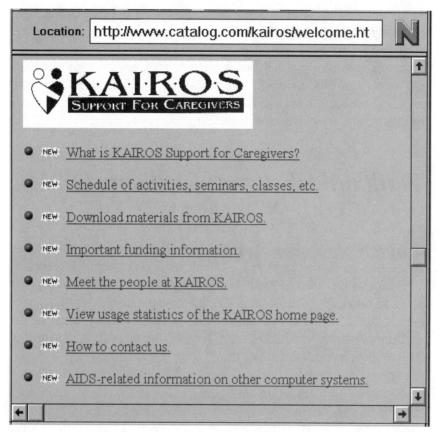

Location: http://www.catalog.com/kairos/welcome.ht

KAIROS
SUPPORT FOR CAREGIVERS

● NEW What is KAIROS Support for Caregivers?

● NEW Schedule of activities, seminars, classes, etc.

● NEW Download materials from KAIROS.

● NEW Important funding information.

● NEW Meet the people at KAIROS.

● NEW View usage statistics of the KAIROS home page.

● NEW How to contact us.

● NEW AIDS-related information on other computer systems.

Kairos supports the people who care for others.

National Institute of Allergy and Infectious Diseases (NIAID)

http://www.niaid.nih.gov

With so many online AIDS resources, it's hard to pick a place to start. You won't go wrong with the NIAID Web page. Here you'll find not only the most up-to-date research information but also popular newsletters, such as AIDS Treatment News, FOCUS (A Guide to Research and Counseling), and AIDS Book Reviews. You'll find links to the AIDS Info BBS, HIVNET, and GPA gopher or Web pages.

You can find information about community resources both in the United States and around the world, and the latest information about existing, emerging, and experimental treatments, including CDC National AIDS Clearinghouse documents. You can read obituaries, book reviews, press releases, speeches, and daily news summaries specifically about AIDS-related issues. Nurses and other healthcare workers will find current recommendations for education, research, and patient care, as well as pointers to other nursing sites online.

National Library of Medicine (NLM)
800-638-8480 (voice)
http://www.nlm.nih.gov/top_level.dir/nlm_online_info.html

The NLM offers free access to three databases devoted to AIDS-related topics. AIDSLINE is an online computer file containing references to AIDS literature in the biomedical, epidemiologic, healthcare administration, oncologic, and social and behavioral sciences fields. The file contains citations (with abstracts when available) of journal articles, monographs, meeting abstracts and papers, government reports, and theses from 1980 to the present. Approximately 1,000 citations are added each month.

You can search the AIDSTRIALS (AIDS Clinical Trials) database for information about AIDS-related studies of experimental treatments conducted under the Food and Drug Administration's investigational new drug regulations. AIDS-TRIALS contains information about clinical trials of agents undergoing evaluation for use against HIV infection, AIDS, and AIDS-related opportunistic diseases, such as pneumocystis carinii pneumonia.

After searching AIDSTRIALS, you can switch to the AIDSDRUGS database and view descriptive information about agents used in clinical trials. It's easy to coordinate searches among the databases since the substance identification number from AIDSDRUGS can be found in the AIDSTRIALS record. Likewise, the protocol numbers from AIDSTRIALS appear in AIDSDRUGS.

The Web page tells how to set up a free account to search these databases 24 hours a day, 7 days a week. The easiest way is using Grateful Med (see chapter

15), which you can also order on the Web page. In addition, the entire AIDS-DRUGS database and AIDSTRIALS records describing open studies are available via FTP from the NLM Publications server (nlmpubs.nlm.nih.gov; login as nlmpubs).

I've been involved in the Internet, or what I'll call the Net, for about five years. It started out quite slowly, mostly sending e-mail to a few colleagues, reading newsgroups every once and a while. Then I began subscribing to a small number of mailing lists. At that point it seemed the world opened up for me.

The mailing list I became most active in is the AIDS mailing list (which is actually a gateway from the Usenet newsgroup sci.med.aids). I was doing AIDS research at the time (and still am), and I found it a valuable resource. I also subscribed to a group called WISENET, which is for women in science, and WMST-L, the Women's Studies List. I realized at that point that the issues I was very interested in, feminism and science and minority health issues, were not covered by any lists or usenet newsgroups I could find. So I decided to create my own groups.

I've mostly enjoyed maintaining mailing lists. Along the way, I was a comoderator for sci.med.aids, which I also enjoyed, but it took quite a bit of time. I've learned that helping to create and maintain the resources available on the Net takes time and effort, but it's very important, in fact crucial to the Net's ongoing survival. I've also helped set up gopher sites and maintain an FTP site for a number of health-related resources.

It's interesting that although the Net is composed of electrical connections between computers, it is in reality made up of connections among individuals. In addition, the Net is always changing and growing, and that's because of the contributions of individuals to it.

Those of us responsible in a broad sense for the health of the population (I include here researchers, as well as health practitioners and policy makers) need access to good information in a timely manner. Scientific and medical knowledge changes at an incredible rate, and our ability to converse with one another over both geographical and disciplinary distance is very important.

I guess my vision is that all of us—researchers, healthcare workers, social service agencies responsible for healthcare (like prenatal care), and people involved in shaping health policy—be involved in dialog and share resources. I think the Internet provides a wonderful opportunity for this vision. I am committed to being a part of the maintenance and expansion of health-related information on the Internet.

Michelle Murrain, Ph.D
http://www.hampshire.edu/Hampshire/ns/html/Murrain.html

Office of the Assistant Secretary for Health (OASH) BBS
202-690-5423

The OASH BBS is the free and publicly accessible electronic bulletin board of the White House Office of the AIDS Policy Coordinator and the U.S. Public Health Service, Office of the Assistant Secretary for Health (OASH). The White House section of the BBS encourages public input on HIV and AIDS issues under consideration. The OASH section of the Public Health Service distributes many AIDS information files, including NLM's AIDS Bibliography, news releases from the NIAID, Federal Register announcements, the CDC's AIDS Daily Summary, and AIDS-related press releases and reports.

Queer Resource Directory (QRD)
gopher://gopher.casti.com/11/gaystuff/QRD/aids

In the AIDS and HIV Information (So Where's Your Red Ribbon?) subdirectory of the QRD, you'll find lots of AIDS information resources, including links to the NIAID gopher server, HIVNET, AIDS BBS, and WHO, in addition to scores of individual news releases, AIDS information from 1992 and 1993, CDC AIDS information, the AIDS Book Review Journal, the AIDS Treatment News-letter, AIDS obituaries, and AIDS conference reports.

University of California, San Francisco (UCSF)
gopher://itsa.ucsf.edu:70/11/

If you're overwhelmed in your search for AIDS information, the UCSF gopher server is a good place to start. From here, you can jump to HIVNET, GPA, NIAID, NLM, CHAT, and several academic AIDS-related gophers that provide additional links to other resources. The UCSF server also provides some documents locally, including clinical practice, quick reference, and consumer guides. Best of all, this gopher serves as a mirror site for Ben Gardiner's AIDS Info BBS database.

– 99 –

Commercial services
CompuServe

go AIDS This directory will point you to every AIDS-related information service offered by CompuServe, including AIDS News Clips, CCML AIDS articles, NORD (which has an AIDS section), Human Sexuality, HealthNet, Health Database Plus, the AMIA Forum, the Education Forum, IQuest, PaperChase, and Information USA.

go AIDSNEWS ($) AIDS News gives you the opportunity to read full-text wire stories about AIDS, HIV infection, and related issues, including Kaposi's sarcoma, dementia, and vaccine development. Political and advocacy stories are also included. AIDS News lists the most recent stories first, which you can read online or mark for later retrieval.

Delphi

go CUSTOM 398 Students That Care is an AIDS awareness and prevention organization that educates the public about the dangers of AIDS and ways to protect yourself from HIV. The group comprises students, teachers, parents, principals, and dignitaries working through the performing arts, television and radio media, and organized events. This custom forum gives interested people an opportunity to share their time and expertise in educating the public about AIDS.

go REF CAIN The Computerized AIDS Information Network (CAIN), located in the Reference and Education directory, provides general information and health agency recommendations related to AIDS. You can search for and request specific documents through I-MED Document Retrieval Service ($$) and CAIN publications ($$), and you can search the database of educational materials (and reviews of them by health educators) located in CAIN itself. You can also take one of several educational quizzes, such as those on AIDS, sexually transmitted diseases, stress, or sexuality. The forum emphasizes news and information but also provides commentaries from individuals posting messages.

GEnie

keyword ARC ($$) GEnie's AIDS Research Center accesses AIDSLINE, a database maintained by the National Library of Medicine. Your search will yield a citation and sometimes an abstract, but not full-text articles. Be aware the NLM has made three databases, including AIDSLINE, available at no charge to the public through its WWW site.

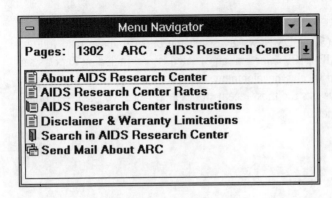

GEnie's AIDS Research Center provides access to AIDSLINE.

7
Cancer

*I*f you or a loved one has been diagnosed with cancer, you'll need information and support. The first places to look are CancerNet and OncoLink, the Internet's two most important sources for cancer information. Two newsgroups (alt.support.cancer and sci.med.diseases.cancer) and a mailing list (Cancer-L) provide forums for general discussion among patients, friends, family members, health care professionals, and researchers. You'll also find sites for information and support for several types of cancer, such as cancer of the breast, brain, and prostate, as well as bone marrow transplants. Finally, most commercial services offer help for cancer patients and their friends and families. Foremost among these services is CompuServe's Cancer Forum, which has informative message boards and databases for most types of cancer.

Throughout cyberspace, you'll notice gopher listings for such renowned research institutions as Dana-Farber Cancer Institute, M.D. Anderson Cancer Center, and Fred Hutchinson Cancer Research Center. Despite the temptation to go first to these sources, be forewarned. There's less than you might expect. These research institutions maintain Internet links mainly so researchers can communicate on the Net; consequently, they have meager online document repositories. Their gophers are handy for locating e-mail addresses of experts or finding dates and times of academic presentations, but there's no need to use their Internet links to reach online cancer resources located elsewhere in cyberspace. It's simpler to go to the other sites directly.

Cancer guides

*CANSEARCH: A Guide to Cancer Resources
(http://access.digex.net/~mkragen/cansearch.html),
Quick Information About Cancer for Patients and Their Families
(http://asa.ugl.lib.umich.edu/chdocs/cancer/
CANCERGUIDE.HTML)*

If you want a wonderfully easy and straightforward tour of online cancer resources, make CANSEARCH your first stop. Marshall Kragen, a cancer survivor and Internet liaison for the National Coalition for Cancer Survivorship, developed CANSEARCH to help the many cancer patients and loved ones seeking online information. Featuring hypertext links to important sites, CANSEARCH is a neatly organized guide to such cancer resources as CancerNet and OncoLink. Before choosing any linked sites, you can read what to expect when you get there. Marshall tells how to find specialized assistance and explains resources he uses to update CANSEARCH (which he does regularly). He also reviews the Coalition's mission, which includes maintaining a survivorship network, serving as a national voice for cancer survivors, and providing support and information about life after a cancer diagnosis.

Judith Gourdji and Susan Hinton have produced an incredible document, Quick Information About Cancer for Patients and Their Families, that will make it easier to decide which of the thousands of available online documents to download and read. This guide reviews major resources of interest to patients and their families, with specific references to breast and prostate cancer. The authors evaluate each document to ensure that it answers the typical questions posed by newly diagnosed cancer patients and their families. Most documents are written for the public rather than for healthcare professionals.

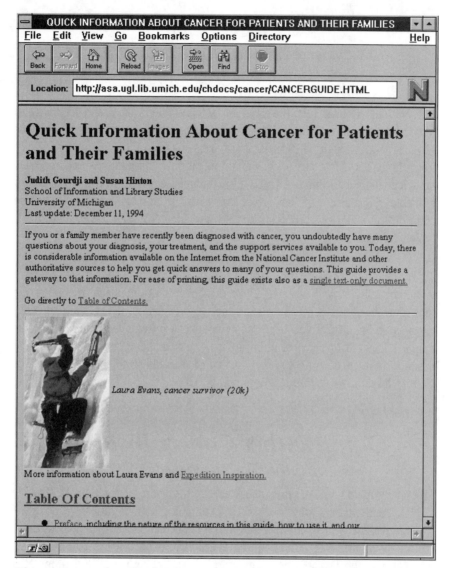

This cancer guide will take you to new heights in your search for help.

CancerNet

cancernet@icicb.nci.nih.gov, gopher.nih.gov,
gopher://gopher.nih.gov:70/11/clin/cancernet,
http://biomed.nus.sg:80/Cancer/welcome.html

The National Cancer Institute's CancerNet is a quick, easy, and free way to obtain cancer information. CancerNet offers information from the NCI's Physician Data Query (PDQ) database, fact sheets on various cancer topics from the NCI's Office of Cancer Communications, and citations and abstracts on selected topics from the CANCERLIT database. Some information is also available in Spanish. The CancerNet Contents List changes monthly to include additions. If you have problems accessing CancerNet, call 1-800-4CANCER (voice) for assistance.

To request information via e-mail, address your message to cancernet @icicb.nci.nih.gov and write HELP in the body of the message to receive the most current contents list. Substitute the word SPANISH if you want the contents list in Spanish. If you have the CancerNet Contents List and want a particular statement or piece of information, enter the code from the list for the desired information. For a complete listing of all gopher and secondary sites for CancerNet documents, request item cn-400030.

Dana-Farber Cancer Institute

gopher://dfci.harvard.edu/

Like many nationally known cancer centers, the Dana-Farber Cancer Institute (DFCI) maintains a gopher server. Unfortunately, it's not much help for the average patient who wants to know more about cancer. The gopher is useful mainly for finding local e-mail addresses and learning about Institute activities. You can use the Dana-Farber gopher to access CancerNet, PDQ, other NIH gophers, and all Harvard University gophers (including the various teaching hospitals affiliated with Harvard Medical School). In addition, the Dana-Farber gopher stores CancerNet information locally in the TechInfo Bulletin Board menu, but we recommend you go directly to CancerNet instead. If you want a list of journal holdings at the Institute, look in the DFCI Libraries subdirectory of the DFCI TechInfo Bulletin Board.

Discussion groups
alt.support.cancer,
Cancer-L (listserv@wvnvm.wvnet.edu), sci.med.diseases.cancer

If you have cancer or know someone with cancer, you can check two Usenet newsgroups (alt.support.cancer and sci.med.diseases.cancer) for answers to almost any question you have. Beyond information, the groups, especially alt.support.cancer, offer emotional support and networking for cancer survivors and their loved ones. The newsgroups welcome physicians and other health-care professionals, cancer researchers, patients (including some truly dedicated cancer survivors), family members, and friends. Typical discussions include the best questions to ask your oncologist, Internet addresses for cancer information, and personal experiences with chemotherapy, radiation therapy, and alternative medicine. Although neither group is moderated, members respond quickly to misinformation and flag advertisements as such. Although members don't generally discourage unconventional therapy, most hold it to the same scientific standard as conventional therapy. Be sure to watch for regular postings of the cancer FAQ, which lists every available online cancer resource.

If you can't access online databases or if you'd rather have the information come to your e-mail address, subscribe to Cancer-L. This highly recommended and very active mailing list discusses diagnosis, treatment, self-examination, and living with cancer. Many physicians and other healthcare professionals respond to questions from list members. You'll find a real sense of community here, with plenty of humor and friendly chatter.

> On March 30, 1992, I was diagnosed with acute myeloid leukemia (AML). Within 24 hours, I received transfusions of packed red blood cells and platelets, had a Groshong catheter surgically implanted in my chest (to allow easy access to a large vein that flows into the heart), had a bone biopsy, and was on chemotherapy.

My wife and I were terrified. We didn't know whether it was possible to survive this type of leukemia or any type of leukemia for that matter. We didn't know the chemotherapy would make me vomit for a week or whether our insurance company would pay the bills.

Fortunately, we had a wonderful family physician, who referred me to an excellent hematologist/oncologist. Still, we had to trust that the doctor was giving me correct information and the proper treatment.

Soon I discovered a Usenet newsgroup, alt.support.cancer, devoted to cancer patients that answered questions I had. On the newsgroup, I read that it was possible to get information on current cancer treatments from the National Cancer Institute (NCI). The NCI confirmed that I had in fact received the best treatment.

For me, the hardest part about being diagnosed with cancer was that I almost completely lost control of my life. I didn't know anything about the diagnosis and treatment of AML. I didn't know what implications this disease would have on the rest of my life. Having knowledge about what was happening and what options were available gave me back some control.

Despite receiving the best treatment and having a relatively good prognosis, I relapsed in January 1993. (AML has a high relapse rate after conventional chemotherapy in adults.) Naively, my wife and I had been sure I was cured. We were not well prepared for the relapse.

The only potentially curative therapy was a bone marrow transplant (BMT), with my brother as the donor. Although a few people in my local support group had received a BMT, none had had an allogeneic one, where the bone marrow comes from someone else, usually a sibling. After posting a message to alt.support.cancer, I was able to "talk" to someone via e-mail about what it was like to have a BMT and what life would be like afterwards. There are many more sources of online information for cancer patients now, including an entire mailing list devoted to BMTs.

I have a fairly unusual kind of cancer. I don't know many people in my city who have this kind of cancer or have had similar treatment. The Internet allows me to exchange information with a much larger group of people. The resources available online are a very valuable source of knowledge. For me, this knowledge has helped to return at least a small sense of control to my life.

Art Flatau

Florida Coalition for Cancer Survivorship
800-816-2744

The Florida Coalition for Cancer Survivorship (FCCS) BBS is devoted to the needs and concerns of cancer survivors, their family members, and oncology healthcare professionals. You'll find the FCCS BBS a friendly place to get cancer information. The interface is smooth—well-organized and easier to navigate than most BBSs—and you can use an online handle. An excellent FAQ on using the BBS is available in the Text Bulletins directory of the Information Menu. Also in the same area is a file that explains the levels of access available

```
Current Topic: Cancer Related message bases

#       Network   Name                          Total  Moderator
1. *!  Local     Cancer Support groups             9
2. *!  Local     My Cancer Story                  13   Drew
3. *!  Local     Where do I get Cancer Info?       2
4. *!  Local     Cancer & Work Related Hassles     7   Isadora Dumpling
5. *!  Local     Death and Dying Issues           32   Isadora Dumpling
6. *!  Local     Living with Cancer Survivors     23   Dances with Weas
7. *!  Internet  alt.support.cancer              202
8. *!  HarmoNet  Cancer Q&A                       24   Hagar
9. *!  Internet  sci.med.diseases.cancer         203
                                                  --
                                                 515

Please Select (1-9) ?) List T)opic List Q)uit:
```

FCCS BBS: The Cancer Connection

The Florida Coalition for Cancer Survivorship BBS offers facts and support.

to members and nonmembers of FCCS. Nonpaying, nonmembers of FCCS can sign on for free but receive less online time with fewer downloads than paying members.

Several message boards address cancer survivorship and issues of interest to oncology healthcare professionals. Highlights of the FCCS BBS include the NCI's PDQ and CANCERLIT databases, hundreds of other cancer-related files and shareware, forums devoted to disease-specific cancer support groups, and a database of tumor images. The FCCS BBS also features the first database of stories written by cancer survivors and their families. In addition, you'll find occasional opinion polls and a live conference area.

National Cancer Center (Tokyo, Japan)
http://www.ncc.go.jp

Once again, the name of this Japanese site sounds more helpful than the services provided, most of which can be reached more quickly and directly in the United States. This server offers CancerNet, Japanese Cancer Research Resources Bank, and National Cancer Center Information, as well as a Cell Line Catalogue and Gene List. Be aware that some documents are typed in Japanese characters.

National Institute for Cancer Research (IST) in Genoa, Italy
http://www.ist.unige.it/

As with the other cancer research center gophers, the IST Web site is most useful to researchers, particularly those working at a molecular level or interested in European databases. Links do exist between IST and every conceivable Internet tool, including most international biomedical gophers. The problem is you have to connect to Italy first and then often backtrack to the United States.

You'll access the American sites faster and less problematically if you go straight to your intended source.

OncoLink

http://www.oncolink.upenn.edu/

While many excellent resources offer cancer information, such as CancerNet and Physician Data Query, OncoLink contains many documents available at these other sites and much more. OncoLink's resources cover almost every type of cancer, treatment, clinical trials, and online patient support service. OncoLink's searching tools are simple to use and yield pages of information. For example, if you need to learn about non-small cell cancer of the lung, one of the most common and insidious lung tumors, a keyword search for *non-small cell lung cancer* will yield almost 50 matches. Clicking on any of the hypertext links will take you to the specific article you want. You could also use OncoLink's Disease Oriented Menus to find Lung Cancer and the submenu of Non-Small Cell or Undifferentiated Cancer.

Using the Internet for medical information

People surfing the Internet for medical information appear to fall into two categories: individuals intent on maintaining or improving their own health and the health of their families, and individuals confronting acute or chronic illness.

Many people with acute, life-threatening illnesses have just experienced the shock of a diagnosis, such as cancer, and have an intense desire to learn the latest information about their disease. They often wish to make contact with others drawn together by their illness. Patients with chronic health problems, such as diabetics, often seek a sense of community with fellow patients to share new findings and methods of coping and to experience a sense of togetherness. Since its creation in March of 1994, I believe OncoLink has touched the lives of millions of people throughout the world.

Providing a sense of community has unique features in cyberspace. Online groups have a special draw, allowing people to share their thoughts with a usually sympathetic audience without leaving their home. The degree of interaction in these communities is under the user's control. The user doesn't have to listen to anyone they don't want to! Online groups also appeal to people who have trouble attending face-to-face meetings because they have a rare disease or have physical limitations or time constraints that make it difficult to travel to local self-help groups.

The Internet provides a powerful set of tools for individuals seeking information. Tools such as World Wide Web browsers are appearing on commercial Internet providers, allowing the casual user to browse medical information throughout the world. A user may begin with an introductory document and find a word, concept, reference—indeed, any point that requires further expansion—underlined as a hypertext key. A simple click of the mouse on this hypertext key fetches more information, be it sound, video, pictures, or more text from somewhere on the Internet. Like picking up a ringing telephone and speaking to the party on the other end, the user is insulated from the "hows" and "whys" of the information gathering process. Simply pressing a button on a WWW menu may unleash powerful search engines to scour multiple sources simultaneously around the world. The result of this search is the equivalent of opening several books to the appropriate page from libraries around the world.

Medical and medically-related information on the Internet enables people to take responsibility for their own health and work in partnership with their healthcare providers. I believe these medical resources will provide the world community with knowledge to take responsibility for their own healthcare. I believe timely and balanced information about healthcare will start a revolution in healthcare.

E. Loren Buhle, Jr. Ph.D.

Physician Data Query (PDQ)

MEDLARS: 800-638-8480 (voice),
PDQ Service Desk: 301-496-7403 (voice),
gopher://uaneuro.uah.ualberta.ca/1

The National Cancer Institute's PDQ is a clinically oriented database about cancer. It was developed to make cancer information widely available to the medical community and the public. PDQ provides state-of-the-art cancer treatment information (including excellent CANCERLIT searching capabilities), research protocols, and directories of physicians and centers providing cancer care. You can access PDQ directly (Grateful Med offers the simplest interface) at $35 per hour between 10 A.M. and 5 P.M. or at $25 per hour at all other times. CompuServe also provides access for an additional fee. Even better, the University of Alberta offers free access to PDQ. You can also find many PDQ documents on OncoLink, the Breast Cancer Information Clearinghouse, CancerNet, and other gopher and Web servers. However, if you decide to search the PDQ database directly, you'll find the sophisticated and well-organized menus a pleasure to use.

Talaria

http://www.stat.washington.edu/TALARIA/TALARIA.html

Talaria, a hypermedia version of the Agency for Healthcare Policy and Research (AHCPR) Guidelines on Cancer Pain, offers both patients and professionals an easy way to move through the complete text while viewing figures, tables, and QuickTime movies. You can start at the Overview or in one of the more specific areas, such as Assessment of Pain in the Patient with Cancer, Pharmacologic Management, Nonpharmacologic Management, Procedure-Related Pain in Adults and Children, Pain in Special Populations, and Monitoring the Quality of Pain Management. Separately, QuickTime movies are also available about chemotherapy-induced oral mucositis, morphine use, and pain in pediatric cancer patients.

Cancer specialty sites
Bone marrow transplants

BMT-Talk (bmt-talk-request@ai.mit.edu),
Day by Day with a Bone Marrow Transplant Patient
(http://www.teleport.com/~tige/cancer/cancer.html)

If you're considering having a bone marrow transplant (BMT), you'll want the latest information on techniques, prognosis, and insurance coverage. One place to turn is an electronic mailing list moderated by Laurel Simmons, a bone marrow transplant recipient. The mailing list is open to anyone who wants to talk about bone marrow transplants. You'll be able to discuss the pros and cons of BMT, exchange information about drug therapy, and share experiences. At least one list member has even posted a diary of BMT experiences.

On the Web, you can read Day by Day with a Bone Marrow Transplant Patient, a comprehensive daily account of one man who had a BMT for multiple myeloma. You'll also find links to other cancer resources.

Other online BMT resources include the BMT Newsletter, Bone Marrow Transplants: A Book of Basics for Patients, and the NCI research report on BMT, all available at the Breast Cancer Information Clearinghouse. The Yale biomedical gopher (see chapter 15, *Searching for medical resources*) also has some issues of the BMT Newsletter (under Organ and Tissue Transplant Information).

Brain tumors
Braintmr (listserv@mitvma.mit.edu)

As with many online resources, the Braintmr list was initiated and remains moderated by a patient, Samantha J. Scolamiero, a brain tumor survivor. Braintmr encourages discussion of topics related to all types of brain tumors, whether benign or malignant. Participants also encourage patients, their supporters, medical professionals, and researchers to share information and experiences.

Breast cancer

*Breast Cancer Information Clearinghouse
(http://nysernet.org/bcic/),
Breast-Cancer (listserv@morgan.ucs.mun.ca)*

If you want to know anything related to breast cancer, check out the Breast Cancer Information Clearinghouse (BCIC). The Clearinghouse offers information obtained through partnership agreements with many organizations, including the American Cancer Society, National Cancer Institute, New York State Department of Health, and National Alliance of Breast Cancer Organizations, as well as many hospitals, libraries, hospices, and nonprofit agencies. The Clearinghouse provides links to OncoLink, CancerNet, and other cancer-related online services. You'll find contact information for regional breast cancer support groups around the country. The server also archives many informative articles about breast cancer and reports on state and federal legislation related to breast cancer, including the President's opinions and policy statements. You can search the Clearinghouse by keyword, check out a weekly update of what's new, and review all of OncoLink's information on breast cancer.

– 113 –

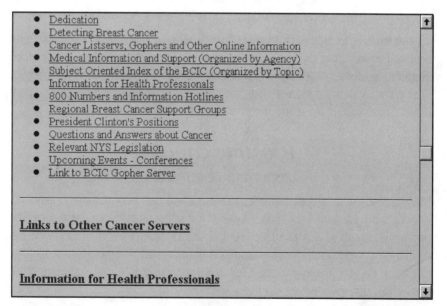

- Dedication
- Detecting Breast Cancer
- Cancer Listservs, Gophers and Other Online Information
- Medical Information and Support (Organized by Agency)
- Subject Oriented Index of the BCIC (Organized by Topic)
- Information for Health Professionals
- 800 Numbers and Information Hotlines
- Regional Breast Cancer Support Groups
- President Clinton's Positions
- Questions and Answers about Cancer
- Relevant NYS Legislation
- Upcoming Events - Conferences
- Link to BCIC Gopher Server

Links to Other Cancer Servers

Information for Health Professionals

The Breast Cancer Information Clearinghouse is a one-stop shopping resource.

To discuss any issue relating to breast cancer, consider subscribing to Breast-Cancer, an unmoderated list open to researchers, physicians, patients, family, and friends of patients. The list doesn't recommend particular therapies, providing instead a broad range of information about options and choices. Members also offer help and insights into the psychosocial management of the disease and provide a forum for venting frustrations about dealing with the disease.

Ovarian cancer
Ovarian-Cancer (listserv@ist01.ferris.edu)

You'll find plenty of warmth and support if you join the Ovarian-Cancer mailing list. Women here keep tabs on each other's treatment and disease status and share their experiences openly—a blessing for newcomers overwhelmed by their recent diagnoses. Patients and professionals exchange opinions and advice in a steady stream of messages.

Power lines and cancer
*http://www.cis.ohio-state.edu/
hypertext/faq/usenet/powerlines-cancer-FAQ*

This extensive six-part FAQ answers questions you might have about the link between power lines (and other sources of electromagnetic fields) and cancer. The FAQ discusses issues ranging from how to use a gaussmeter to how power lines affect real-estate values. The FAQ also reviews most major studies published to date about the association between power lines and cancer.

Prostate cancer
alt.support.cancer.prostate

Members of the active alt.support.cancer.prostate newsgroup share their experiences with prostate cancer and seek information about the latest scientific findings in the diagnosis and treatment of this disease. They discuss the merits of different surgical approaches and the implications of laboratory tests that track the spread of the cancer. Online membership is diverse and includes physicians and even wives who talk openly about sex and orgasm after their husbands' radical prostatectomies.

Commercial services

While all the commercial services offer oncology resources in their general medical areas (see chapter 5, *General health information*), only CompuServe devotes an entire forum to cancer information and support.

CompuServe

go CANCER ($) CompuServe's Cancer Forum is the best place for information and support, 24 hours a day, 7 days a week. It's like the OncoLink of commercial services, although on a reduced scale. The support staff includes members of the Forum and the Kansas City Cancer Hotline. Message sections and libraries cover most types of cancer, including breast, uterine, cervical, ovarian, prostate, testicular, head and neck, lung, bladder and kidney, brain and spinal cord, skin (including melanoma), bone and soft tissues (including sarcoma), gastrointestinal, blood-related (including leukemia), pediatric, and rare types. Information about insurance issues, political action, hospice care, nutrition, and research is also available. In the forum's libraries, you'll find software, PDQ files (both patient and physician versions), and hundreds of fact sheets and other documents related to cancer. In the message sections, you can discuss cancer-related topics and direct questions to people who are battling the disease. Finally, you can join others in the conference area for seminars and informal chats.

8

Specific diseases and disorders

*T*his chapter provides a slice of what's available for the dozens of diseases and medical conditions discussed online. All subject areas are listed alphabetically. We list some conditions by disease name (diabetes, Lyme disease, hepatitis), while others are clustered by organ system (heart disease, gastrointestinal diseases, muscle disorders).

If you don't find the medical condition you want, check other chapters in this book. For example, we discuss Alzheimer's disease in chapter 9, *Neurologic disorders,* and endometriosis in the women's health section of chapter 12, *Patient groups.* Computer use-related injuries (carpal tunnel syndrome, repetitive strain injury, electromagnetic field radiation), of particular interest to frequent online users, are discussed in chapter 11, *From teeth to toes.* If you don't find a topic listed in this chapter or the index, then read chapter 15, *Searching for medical resources,* to learn how to find the latest online resources. Finally, keep in mind that the best way to keep informed of the latest online and offline medical resources is to read FAQs and join newsgroups or Fidonet conferences related to your interests.

Allergies

alt.med.allergy

Whether the problem is food, pets, or pollen, individuals with allergies can turn to this active Usenet newsgroup. Discussions center on ways people cope with their allergies. Topics range from medications to allergy shots to other therapies. Participants review books, post medical information from journals, and share stories about dealing with their allergies. Parents of children with allergies will find additional help in the misc.kids.health and misc.kids newsgroups (see chapter 12, *Patient groups*), which maintain an Allergies/Asthma FAQ. For specific information on food allergies, you can check the International Food Information Council (http://ificinfo.health.org/allergy.htm).

Aneurysms

http://www.cc.columbia.edu:80/~mdt1/./

Patients with aneurysms, balloon-like swellings of blood vessels, often feel as though they're carrying a time bomb. If you, a friend, or family member has an aneurysm, you'll find Dr. M. David Tilson's Aneurysm Information Project an excellent source of information. This Web site offers an Aneurysm FAQ, lectures, papers, references, bibliographies, and patient stories. The FAQ focuses on abdominal aortic aneurysms, although some of the information is applicable to brain aneurysms. The FAQ and other documents address the importance of early detection, prevention of rupture and other complications, and repair of aneurysms. Also available are the American Aneurysm Foundation mission statement and details about the University of Vermont's Aneurysm Prevention Project and the University of Iowa's Aneurysm Imaging Project.

Arthritis

*alt.support.arthritis, Arthritis Foundation
(ftp://ftp.netcom.com/pub/ar/arthritis/),
Arthritis-L (listproc@showme.missouri.edu), misc.health.arthritis,
Sjögren's Syndrome Foundation Inc. (http://www.w2.com/ss.html),
SS (listserv@vmd.cso.uiuc.edu)*

Your options for information about arthritis include newsgroups, mailing lists, an FTP site, a gopher, and a Web site. The newsgroups alt.support.arthritis and misc.health.arthritis, and the discussion group Arthritis-L (which includes postings from alt.support.arthritis), offer support for arthritis patients and helpful information from physicians and researchers who deal with the disease. In misc.health.arthritis especially, you'll learn about new clinical trials and other basic science information. A FAQ is also available. Finally, you'll find literature posted by the Arthritis Foundation available through FTP.

In addition to rheumatoid and osteoarthritis, the newsgroups and mailing lists discuss lupus, Reiter's Syndrome, and Sjögren's syndrome (SS). In fact, if dry eyes, a dry mouth, or a dry nose accompany your arthritis, you could have SS and might want to investigate the Sjögren's Syndrome Foundation Web site for more information. You can also subscribe to the SS mailing list. For information about arthritis related to Lyme disease, you can read about LymeNet later in this chapter.

> The diseases I work with range from the very common, such as rheumatoid arthritis and ankylosing spondylitis, to the very rare. While most of these diseases are not curable, they are quite treatable. I found it useful to learn about the different ways some of these diseases are treated in other parts of the world. I often find myself talking on the Internet to colleagues about interesting people and problems I have encountered.

When people ask for help, it's difficult to give specific advice without knowing all the details and examining the person. I'm able to clear up misconceptions about some of the rheumatic diseases and point people in the right direction. Sometimes a person's symptoms match another disease, and I will mention the possibility. Another area that I find I have been commenting on is drugs and drug side effects—particularly for some of the more potent disease-modifying therapies.

Kam Shojania, M.D., F.R.C.P.C.

Asthma

alt.support.asthma; National Heart, Lung, and Blood Institute (NHLBI) (gopher://gopher.nhlbi.nih.gov/)

The alt.support.asthma newsgroup provides a forum for the discussion of asthma: its symptoms, causes, and treatment. The group maintains an excellent general information FAQ that includes personal experiences, suggestions, and practical information about asthma and other respiratory disorders. There's also an asthma medications FAQ and a Reading/Resource List. In the newsgroup, you can pick up a variety of tips, such as which air filters work best for most people, and learn about offline resources. You can also turn to misc.kids.health for additional information. You can also access the NHLBI gopher for information from the National Asthma Education and Prevention Program (in the Education Programs and Activities directory).

Autism

listserv@sjuvm.bitnet, bit.listserv.autism

You can share your experiences with autism either by subscribing to the mailing list or reading the bit.listserv.autism newsgroup. Both groups provide a forum for those affected by the disorder, including families, teachers of autistic children, and caregivers. The Autism FAQ (see appendix C) explains how to join the discussion group, thoroughly reviews autism, and includes a glossary, bibliography, and list of organizations and services.

Balance disorders

Johns Hopkins Center for Hearing and Balance
(http://www.bme.jhu.edu/labs/chb/),
University of Michigan Medical Center
(http://www.anes.med.umich.edu/oto/index.html)

If you have trouble with balance, one resource is the Vestibular Testing Center of the University of Michigan Medical Center's Department of Otolaryngology. The Center offers vestibular rehabilitation that trains the patient's central nervous system to compensate for balance problems. On the Web page, you'll find a document explaining how vestibular rehabilitation works, possible outcomes following treatment, and criteria for patient selection.

The Johns Hopkins Center for Hearing and Balance also maintains a Web page on this topic. The goal of the Center is to perform basic and clinical research about auditory (hearing) and vestibular (balance) function, train basic and clinical investigators, and disseminate research results and relevant information to the medical community and the public. At the Center's Web page, you'll be able to read recent research results, case studies from the weekly vestibular rounds, test your understanding of the vestibular system (directed more toward clinicians than patients), find a glossary, and review a FAQ about dizziness and the vestibular system.

Chronic fatigue syndrome

alt.med.cfs, bit.listserv.cfs.newsletter,
Cathar-M (listserv@sjuvm.stjohns.edu),
CFS/CFIDS/ME (http://www.astro.uva.nl/fluks/me.html),
CFS-L (cfs-l-request@list.nih.gov)

Anyone interested in learning more about chronic fatigue syndrome (also known as chronic fatigue immune deficiency syndrome or myalgic encephalomyelitis, and sometimes associated with chronic Epstein-Barr virus) will find more help online than almost anywhere else. Roger Burns, a contributor to many CFS resources, is moderator of alt.med.cfs. He has categorized postings by the type of information provided, helping group members more easily find what they need. You can also participate in this newsgroup via the mailing list CFS-L.

Catharsis, a monthly newsmagazine, offers personal, medical, and functional support to people with chronic fatigue immune deficiency syndrome (CFIDS), their spouses and family members, and those who share an interest in CFIDS and related problems.

The CFS/ME Computer Networking Project, comprised of CFS section leaders from major computer networks, operates the CFS newswire service and facilitates communication with various CFS sites. To find out about the latest CFS internet resources, send GET CFS NET-HELP or GET CFS-NET TXT as an e-mail message to listserv@sjuvm.stjohns.edu. Roger Burns, a founding member of the CFS/ME Computer Networking Project, notes that "the network resources available about CFS will help doctors looking for advice from their professional peers about treatment and diagnosis; people looking for quick sources of CFS medical news; patients looking for information, support, and advice about how to deal with this illness; and severely ill patients who are disabled and who cannot attend the usual support group meetings or gather other needed information."

Finally, the CFS/CFIDS/ME Web site offers in one convenient location links to just about every CFS-related online resource, including Catharsis, CFS-File, CFS-L/Usenet alt.med.cfs, CFS-News, CFS Village (Australia), CFS-WIRE, CFS-WWW (Canada), Fibrom-L/Usenet alt.med.fibromyalgia, Gulf War Resource pages, LymeNet Newsletter, and several European resources. Digging through some of the directories will lead you to additional useful online resources including several freenets, mainly in Canada.

In 1985, I became ill with a mysterious ailment that confounded the best of physicians. After a very thorough examination, it was determined that I was suffering from a chronic, viral syndrome of unknown etiology. I spent the first years of my illness bed-ridden and isolated. It was a traumatic existence for a formerly outgoing and energetic young woman of 22. The next years I fared somewhat better and even tried to return to college on a limited basis. I wasn't successful.

Around Christmas, 1990, I was given a modem by a friend. Little did I know this device would alter my life dramatically.

The first thing I found using my modem was that I could connect to commercial services and chat live with people around the country. Second, I discovered local bulletin boards, where people in my own community discussed a wide variety of subjects. I became aware that this modem was helping me find the social and intellectual interaction I had been lacking.

I also became involved with GEnie. Interested in my illness, now acknowledged as chronic fatigue syndrome (CFS) by the Centers for Disease Control, I looked for information, resources, and support. I found the support in the form of other sufferers who had collected in a small area within GEnie's Medical BBS. By the next year, the CFS group moved to GEnie's DisAbilities area, where we found a lot of support from others who had dealt with many aspects of disability—from medical issues to legal concerns to coping skills. I went from running the CFS category to being asked to become Assistant Systems Operator of the disability area.

Finding myself in a position of responsibility was an incredible boost to my self-esteem. Every time I did a job well I felt a certain worthiness and a sense of "can-do." It wasn't much later that I joined other networkers using the Internet and various commercial services, and we combined efforts to spread support, medical information, and news across the globe.

Since that time I have finished my B.A. in Technical Writing from home and am currently studying for my Masters at the New School for Social Research in New York via modem. I am also in the process of starting my own communications company.

What began as a quest for medical information resulted in my finding the prosthetic device that has made vocation, education, and social interaction available to me even when my illness, after 10 years, leaves me home-bound. The knowledge, esteem, and possibilities that are mine today are a direct result of this technology. What better medicine?

Molly Holzschlag
Tucson, Arizona

Cystic fibrosis

Cystic-L (listserv@yalevm.cis.yale.edu)

The Cystic-L discussion group focuses on new medical advances and possible therapeutic and nutritional treatments for cystic fibrosis. The forum also allows patients to vent feelings about frustrating encounters, biases, and other challenges posed by this disease.

Diabetes

alt.support.diabetes.kids, Diabetes Friends Action Network Newsletter (belve@delphi.com), Diabetes Knowledgebase (http://www.biostat.wisc.edu/diaknow/index.htm), Diabetic (listserv@lehigh.edu), misc.health.diabetes, National Institute of Diabetes and Digestive and Kidney Diseases (http://www.niddk.nih.gov/), Type-One (listserv@netcom.com)

You'll find several online resources for all types of diabetes. Good starting points are two Usenet newsgroups (misc.health.diabetes and alt.support.diabetes.kids), which offer support and information exchange to patients, their families, and healthcare professionals. Misc.health.diabetes members discuss issues of diabetes management (Type I, Type II, and gestational), including diet, activities, medicine schedules, blood glucose control, software, exercise, and medical breakthroughs. Helpful FAQs are posted on the newsgroups and at Diabetes Knowledgebase. Not surprisingly, alt.support.diabetes.kids offers information sharing, emotional support, and guidance aimed specifically at families whose children have diabetes mellitus. The group might split to allow teens with diabetes to form a separate subgroup.

Using just e-mail, you can subscribe to the very active Diabetic discussion group, the main mailing list for diabetics or those with an interest in the disease. The list carries about 60 to 80 messages per day. If you prefer a single collective posting, you can convert your subscription to digest form. Another discussion group is Type-One, which split off from the Diabetic group to focus on Type I diabetes, also known as insulin-dependent diabetes. This mailing list serves more as a support group than a source of medical information, with members sharing experiences and advice. You can also subscribe to an electronic newsletter full of articles and patient stories from the Diabetes Friends Action Network on Delphi.

> I am an editor of a magazine for young diabetics in Croatia. I have been using Internet services for only five months, and I am in a whole new field of communications. I posted my article as a test only, but I received three replies.
>
> One boy from the U.S. who is on an insulin pump promised to send me some information about using an insulin pump every day. Here in Croatia, it is not very usual to see people on pumps, because people do not know very much about them.
>
> I would appreciate hearing from anyone who has information to send me that will be useful for young diabetics.
>
> Antun Paulin
> Antun.Paulin@public.srce.hr

Established at the University of Wisconsin Medical School by Dr. Donald Lehn, Diabetes Knowledgebase provides answers to many of the questions you have about both Type I (insulin-dependent or childhood onset) and Type II (noninsulin-dependent or adult onset) diabetes mellitus. Also available at the Web site are FAQs; information about diabetic newsgroups; the Diabetic Friends Action Network Newsletter; a glossary of diabetes-related terms; a glycemic index page; stories for children about dealing with diabetes; and connections to the American, Canadian, and British Diabetes Associations and the Juvenile Diabetes Foundation. Dr. Lehn announces new additions to the Web site through postings to the diabetes newsgroups and mailing lists. Whether you've had diabetes a few months or most of your life, you'll find Diabetes Knowledgebase a great source for up-to-date information.

Finally, like many institutes at the NIH, the National Institute of Diabetes and Digestive and Kidney Diseases (NIDDK) has launched its own Web page. At the NIDDK you'll find a diabetes dictionary, an overview of diabetes, materials on complications of diabetes, U.S. diabetes statistics, professional and voluntary diabetes organizations, and information about the Diabetes Control and Complications Trial. From the NIDDK Web page, you can jump to other institutes at the NIH.

Among people with chronic illnesses, those with diabetes are in a unique situation. If given the right information, they can personally control their medical condition and directly influence the impact it has on their lives. By carefully monitoring their blood sugar levels and adjusting their insulin, hypoglycemic agent, diet, exercise, and daily activities accordingly, they can maintain virtually normal blood sugar levels and thus prevent or at least delay the onset of the long-term complications associated with diabetes.

The University of Wisconsin Medical School's Diabetes Knowledgebase was created to assist in providing diabetes-related information to the world community in an effort to enhance the lives of individuals with diabetes. By utilizing the recently developed World Wide Web client/server capabilities of the Internet, it is possible to provide diabetes-related information to the more than 20 million Internet users, 5% of whom are estimated to have diabetes. Since the Diabetes Knowledgebase was put online in October of 1994, more than 10,000 people visit each month, even though its existence has been disseminated only through word-of-mouth and a few announcements in the Usenet newsgroup misc.health.diabetes.

Although we have received many positive responses from people who have accessed the Diabetes Knowledgebase, the truly remarkable aspect of these responses has not been their number or content but rather their geographic origin. We have received comments from users in England, France, Germany, Norway, South Africa, Israel, Australia, Canada, Belgium, Brazil, Poland, China, New Zealand, Mexico, Spain, Italy, and Japan. This clearly shows that the World Wide Web is aptly named.

A long-term goal of the Diabetes Knowledgebase is to develop a comprehensive, educational resource to be used by doctors, certified diabetic educators, nutritionists, and people with diabetes. An immediate goal is to develop a series of educational "units" geared toward particular audiences, such as the parents of young diabetic children, diabetic teenagers, young adults, and caregivers. With this information provided on the Internet, people worldwide will have easy access to it—not merely those who happen to live close to a major medical center.

Donald A. Lehn, Ph.D.

Down's syndrome

bit.listserv.down-syn, Down-Syn (listserv@vm1.nodak.edu),
Down Syndrome WWW Page (http://www.nas.com/downsyn/)

A Usenet newsgroup, mailing list, and Fidonet conference all provide much useful information and support for individuals and families concerned about Down's syndrome. In these groups, members share their thoughts, frustrations, hopes, and prayers. Not surprisingly, many messages on Down-Syn relate to medications and medical problems as well as testing and developmental issues. On the mailing list you'll also be able to keep track of online resources and legislative and advocacy issues.

In addition, Tracey Finch has created the Down Syndrome Web Page, which includes several articles, poems, and essays; a book list; and links to the Arc (which has its own excellent Down's syndrome FAQ), Our Kids, and Attention Deficit Disorder Web pages. You'll also find the Down's Syndrome Preventive Medical Checklist compiled by the Ohio/Western PA Down's Syndrome Network. The Checklist is especially useful for tracking particular medical problems that affect Down's syndrome children and adults. With the help of the Down-Syn community, the Down Syndrome Web Page has become a dynamic resource for anyone seeking information and support.

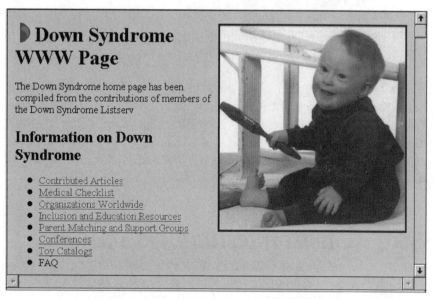

Families looking for support can turn to the Down Syndrome WWW Page.

Endocrine disorders

*National Institute of Diabetes and Digestive
and Kidney Diseases (http://www.niddk.nih.gov/)*

The NIDDK Web page (described earlier for diabetes) also provides information on other endocrine disorders, including Addison's disease, Cushing's syndrome, and familial multiple endocrine neoplasia. You can check here for fact sheets on specific endocrine diseases or watch the sci.med newsgroup to see if there are any new newsgroups or mailing lists that address your topic of interest.

Fibrositis/fibromyalgia

*alt.med.fibromyalgia,Fibrom-L (listserv@vmd.cso.uiuc.edu),
USA Fibrositis Association (http://www.w2.com/fibro1.html)*

The USA Fibrositis Association offers a Web page to help fibrositis patients. Concisely written documents address the pain of fibrositis, living with fibrositis, finding local help, and joining the Fibrositis Association. The Association emphasizes self-education and the benefits of a positive attitude in learning how to modify activity to adjust to the condition.

Fibrom-L, an active, unmoderated list, offers a forum for researchers, physicians, patients, family and friends of patients, and other interested people. Participants post helpful information, answer questions, share conversation and humor, and give tremendous support to all who join. Multiple FAQs are available as well. The Usenet newsgroup alt.med.fibromyalgia offers another site for reading and responding to Fibrom-L messages.

Gastrointestinal diseases
alt.support.crohn-colitis, alt.support.ostomy,
Celiac (listserv@sjuvm.stjohns.edu), Crohn's Disease/Ulcerative
Colitis/IBS server (http://qurlyjoe.bu.edu/cduchome.html),
National Institute of Diabetes and Digestive and Kidney Diseases
(http://www.niddk.nih.gov/)

If you have almost any type of gastrointestinal problem, you'll find tremendous support from the Usenet newsgroup alt.support.crohn-colitis, which draws people with ulcerative colitis, Crohn's disease, irritable bowel syndrome, and other related disorders. Participants discuss various treatment and management techniques, healthcare providers, related illnesses, and their everyday struggles with gastrointestinal disease. Alt.support.crohn-colitis has three terrific FAQs—inflammatory bowel disease (IBD), irritable bowel syndrome (IBS), and info-resources—which also are available on the Web pages described later in this section. The FAQs, posted biweekly, explain diagnostic tests, drug therapies, surgical options, dietary recommendations, and techniques for preventing symptom flare-ups. You might also want to tune-in to live conference discussion at the #crohns IRC channel.

As the name indicates, alt.support.ostomy provides support for anyone living with an ostomy. Although initially not very active, the group has a few dedicated members who are working hard to spread the word about this Usenet group.

The Celiac list serves those interested in celiac disease, dermatitis herpetiformis, gluten intolerance, wheat allergy, and other types of food intolerances such as casein or lactose. If you join this open, unmoderated discussion, you'll learn about the latest scientific research, what food is gluten-free, how to eat out, and how to cope.

Bill Robertson's Crohn's Disease/Ulcerative Colitis/IBS Web Pages bring a number of resources together. This site provides information and encouragement to patients through links to various FAQs, references, and postings from those who have visited the page. You'll find the three FAQs discussed earlier, information about the I.B. Details newsletter, links to the alt.support.crohns-colitis and alt.support.ostomy newsgroups (and their archives), and "some butt-headed humor."

Finally, you can find information on digestive diseases at the NIDDK server. Look for the Consensus Development Conference report on the link between helicobacter pylori and peptic ulcer disease. You'll also find patient information

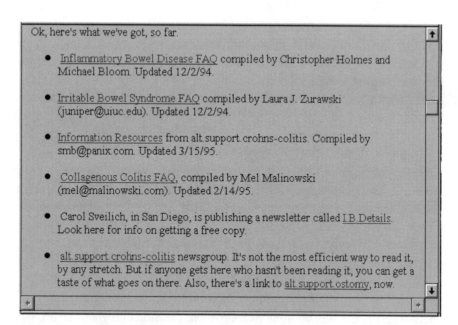

Ok, here's what we've got, so far.

- Inflammatory Bowel Disease FAQ compiled by Christopher Holmes and Michael Bloom. Updated 12/2/94.

- Irritable Bowel Syndrome FAQ compiled by Laura J. Zurawski (juniper@uiuc.edu). Updated 12/2/94.

- Information Resources from alt.support.crohns-colitis. Compiled by smb@panix.com. Updated 3/15/95.

- Collagenous Colitis FAQ, compiled by Mel Malinowski (mel@malinowski.com). Updated 2/14/95.

- Carol Sveilich, in San Diego, is publishing a newsletter called I.B. Details. Look here for info on getting a free copy.

- alt.support.crohns-colitis newsgroup. It's not the most efficient way to read it, by any stretch. But if anyone gets here who hasn't been reading it, you can get a taste of what goes on there. Also, there's a link to alt.support.ostomy, now.

Most disease-related Web pages include FAQs, archives, and other useful documents.

on constipation, heartburn, hemorrhoids, lactose intolerance, and voluntary digestive disease organizations.

Heart disease

American Heart Association (gopher://gopher.amhrt.org), Cardiology Compass (http://osler.wustl.edu/ ~murphy/cardiology/compass.html), The Heart: A Virtual Exploration (http://sln.fi.edu/biosci/heart.html), National Heart, Lung, and Blood Institute (gopher://gopher.nhlbi.nih.gov/)

The American Heart Association (AHA) offers a gopher server, while a Web site and FTP access under construction are probably available now. The AHA site offers general information about the organization (including volunteer opportunities and research programs), legislative updates, community and educational programs, heart-healthy information, patient support groups, scientific publications, conferences and meetings, news releases, and fact sheets with biostatistical information.

To learn more about your heart and its relationship to your health, you can go to The Heart: A Virtual Exploration, which is located at the Franklin Institute Science Museum's Web site. You can peruse a table of contents or use the Web's search function to explore the exhibit. The site also provides recommended resource materials, activities, and a glossary.

Cardiology Compass will take you almost anywhere you might want to go for cardiology information. Links include the American College of Cardiology, the American Heart Association, the Cardiovascular Disease Network, Heart Sounds, the Aneurysm Information Project, the Cardiac Prevention Research Center, the UCSF Division of General Internal Medicine (hypertension management), the NHLBI Gopher, nutrition and cardiovascular bibliographies, and the Cardiac Arrhythmia Advisory System.

The National Heart, Lung, and Blood Institute (NHLBI) offers a gopher server that's regularly updated with information about education programs and initiatives, research grant opportunities, scientific meeting reports and summaries, task force panel reports, and advisory council updates. The NHLBI oversees research on cholesterol, high blood pressure, heart failure, coronary heart disease, arrhythmias, cardiopulmonary dysfunction, artificial heart and other cardiovascular technologies, asthma, smoking, strokes, blood disorders (such as sickle cell anemia), and many other related conditions. The Institute also provides information of special interest to women and minorities.

Hepatitis

Hepv-L (listserv@sjuvm.stjohns.edu)

With postings from Croatia, Canada, Germany, the United States, and other countries around the world, Geff Thorpe's Hepv-L mailing list offers an international symposium for hepatitis information and support. Hepv-L is an unmoderated discussion group for people diagnosed with chronic hepatitis, as well as physicians, nurses, family members, and others concerned about the illness. The group shares personal stories and suggestions for keeping spirits high, exchanges medical and scientific information, and discusses daily management concerns.

Kidney and urologic disease

Renalnet (gopher://ns.gamewood.net/11/renalnet/),
National Institute of Diabetes and Digestive Diseases
(http://www.niddk.nih.gov/)

Renalnet is a forum for communication and information exchange within the nephrology community. You can reach it through both a gopher server and a Web link. Renalnet offers educational material, research information, conference agendas, and product information. Also available is the full text of the NIH Consensus Development Conference on Dialysis Morbidity and Mortality. You can read stories of kidney transplants, archives of *MedNews*, and the *Morbidity and Mortality Weekly Report*. You can also access the Usenet transplantation newsgroup and links to other online resources.

The NIDDK Web page offers another option for finding information on kidney and urologic disorders. You'll find information on end-stage renal disease, kidney stones, urinary tract infections, interstitial cystitis, and prostate enlargement.

Lyme disease
LymeNet (gopher://gopher.lymenet.org:70/1),
LymeNet-L (listserv@lehigh.edu)

The Lyme Disease Network of NJ, Inc., a nonprofit organization dedicated to disseminating information about Lyme disease, maintains the LymeNet gopher server with medical, legal, support, and advocacy resources. You'll find the full text of court cases and public-opinion articles in addition to guidelines for diagnosis, treatment, and management of the disease. The gopher also carries government documents, notes from Lyme disease scientific conferences and meetings, and even some humor. When you first access the gopher, read the comprehensive LymeNet Resource Guide, which provides an overview of Lyme disease, information about LymeNet, a list of online Lyme disease resources, and subscription information for the bimonthly LymeNet Newsletter. By now, the LymeNet Mailing List might be linked with the misc.health.lyme-disease newsgroup.

Muscle disorders
alt.support.musc-dystrophy, CMTnet
(http://www.ultranet.com/~smith/CMTnet.html),
MD-List (MD-List-Request@data.basix.com), MD-List Archives
(gopher://link.tsl.texas.gov:70/1m/.dir/libmail.dir/.files/zmdlist),
Muscular Dystrophy Ireland (http://www.iol.ie/~coreilly/mdi.html)

You'll find that alt.support.musc-dystrophy covers a wide range of muscular disorders, including muscular dystrophy, myotonic dystrophy, spinal muscular atrophy, myasthenia gravis, and myotubular myopathy. Although you might find that you're the only participant dealing with a particular disorder, the group freely shares support and available information.

The MD-List, created for parents, family and friends, and caregivers, provides support and encourages sharing information and advice. In Ireland, you'll find a growing Web page with information and resources for both muscular dystrophy and Charcot-Marie Tooth disease (with a link to CMTnet), as well as links to many disability-related resources.

You'll find more information about Charcot-Marie Tooth, a neuromuscular disease, on an excellent series of Web pages. CMTnet offers a tutorial about the disease, a list of CMT toxic substances, information about CMT support organizations, and reviews of genetic research, biochemistry, electrical stimulation, orthopedics, and orthotics. CMTnet also provides links for resources for carpal tunnel syndrome, which resembles CMT in the hands. You can also join a CMT e-mail discussion list, MD-List, and several Usenet newsgroups.

Polio

alt.support.post-polio, Polio (listserv@sjuvm.stjohns.edu),
Polio Survivors Page (http://www.eskimo.com/~dempt/polio.html)

While many consider polio a disease of the past, some still struggle with its aftermath. The Usenet newsgroup alt.support.post-polio offers polio survivors and their families, friends, and healthcare providers an opportunity to make friends and share support. You'll read about how to find local support groups and how to manage associated disabilities. You'll also learn about the latest medical developments in the field. One active group member, Robert Mauro, started and maintains the Polio mailing list, an unmoderated forum for discussion and support among persons with polio or post-polio syndrome. Members discuss the effects of polio, various medical treatments, pain management and other challenges, and new drugs and other therapies. Both the newsgroup and the list share postings. If you want to join live conversations, go to the #polio IRC channel.

Another active newsgroup member, Tom Dempsey, maintains the Polio Survivors Page, which provides links to other online polio resources and articles. You'll find the full text of Atlanta Post Polio Association Newsletters, nontechnical articles (patient experiences, commentaries, and general information), an information packet, post-polio medical articles and bibliographies, Social Security

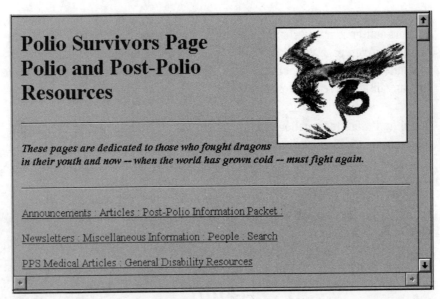

Polio Survivors Page
Polio and Post-Polio
Resources

These pages are dedicated to those who fought dragons
in their youth and now -- when the world has grown cold -- must fight again.

Announcements : Articles : Post-Polio Information Packet :

Newsletters : Miscellaneous Information : People : Search

PPS Medical Articles : General Disability Resources

Polio survivors can come together online.

information, and topographical maps of the polio Type 1 and Type 3 viruses. The page also provides links to other polio online resources, disability resources, the Guide to Emotional Support Resources, and other medical resources. Not surprisingly, early in its life the page had more than 3,000 visits in a one-month period.

Rare disorders

National Organization for Rare Disorders
(http://www.w2.com/nord1.html),
Rare-Dis (listserv@sjuvm.stjohns.edu)

If you struggle to find information and support for a rare disease, check out the Web page for the National Organization for Rare Disorders (NORD). Their mission is three-fold. They seek to educate both the public and medical profession about the existence, diagnosis, and treatment of rare disorders; to act as a clearinghouse for information about rare disorders; and to network families with similar disorders for mutual support. If you want to research

NORD's databases directly, you can access them through CompuServe, as described later in this chapter. At the Web site you can scan a listing of rare diseases to find the one you're looking for. You can then order a $5 reprint that describes the rare disorder, its symptoms, cause, affected population, standard and investigational treatments, and additional resources for more information. Finally, you can check local freenets and BBSs for discussions of rare disorders, subscribe to the Rare-Dis mailing list, and tag the Fidonet conference Rare_Condition to meet others facing the same ordeal.

Sleep disorders
alt.support.sleep-disorders, Sleep Medicine Home Page
(http://www.cloud9.net/~thorpy),
SNORE (http://www.access.digex.net/~faust/sldord/)

Whether you have simple insomnia or more serious disorders such as sleep apnea, narcolepsy, night terrors, or sleep walking, you'll want to check out alt.support.sleep-disorders. To get started, read the group's excellent FAQ, prepared with assistance from the National Sleep Foundation. Then read messages from members who share their experiences with continuous positive airway pressure (CPAP), sleep studies, various medications, and other methods of improving sleep duration and quality.

For more in-depth information about sleep disorders, you'll want to go to Dr. Michael Thorpy's Sleep Medicine Home Page. Here you'll find information for patients and links to other resources for more on sleep physiology, sleep research, government-supported programs, and sleep-related professional organizations and associations. You can also read about mailing lists (mainly for healthcare professionals) and newsgroups. Other sleep-related topics covered at this site include enuresis (bedwetting), obstructive sleep apnea, infant sleep apnea (including an NIH Consensus Development Conference statement), sudden infant death syndrome, sleep disorders in older adults, and use of medications to promote sleep. Organizations represented at this site include the National Sleep Foundation, the American Sleep Apnea Association, the Narcolepsy Network, the Restless Legs Syndrome Foundation, American Sleep Disorders Association, the Sleep Research Association, the European Sleep Research Society, and the World Federation of Sleep Research Societies.

The SNORE (Sleep Apnoea Online Resource For Education) Web page, maintained by Doug Linder, provides information on obstructive sleep apnea and other sleep disorders. Included are files that offer general information about sleep apnea, beds, snoring, apnea in children, and (to a lesser extent) other sleep disorders. You'll also find tips on living with obstructive sleep apnea and a sleep disorder bibliography, as well as links to other sleep resources and documents. A Sleep Apnoea FAQ is currently under construction.

Tinnitus
alt.support.tinnitus

Do you often hear buzzing or ringing in your ears? You might want to join alt.support.tinnitus, where you can meet other people who suffer tinnitus from Ménière's disease, hyperacusis, and other disorders. Participants comment on various treatments, including surgical and drug therapy, discuss possible causes or triggers, and offer help finding specialists. This newsgroup also posts, monthly, a very comprehensive and quite lengthy Tinnitus FAQ, which you can also find on the Web at http://www.cccd.edu/faq/tinnitus.html.

Commercial services

All the commercial online services provide information and support for many individual diseases and conditions. We've listed the forums that specifically address a single disorder or cluster of disorders. If you don't see the topic you're looking for here, check the broader health forum discussion groups and library files. For example, on GEnie try the Medical RoundTable, and on Prodigy the Health BB and the Medical Support BB. America Online covers many diseases in their Better Health & Medical Forum, as does e•World in Living Well and CompuServe in the Health and Fitness Forum.

CompuServe

go DIABETES ($) The Diabetes and Hypoglycemia Forum brings together people with a common interest in diabetes, hypoglycemia, and related chronic metabolic disorders. This very active forum encourages members to tell about their personal experiences (so that others can learn from them), share information, ask questions, voice opinions, and offer support. The libraries and message sections share the same title and number, and include the following topics: Insulin & Oral Medications, Parenting Issues, Diet & Exercise, Complications, Paraphernalia (Mechanical, Electronic, Computer), Insulin Pumps, Pregnancy & Sex, the International Family of Diabetics (IFD), Ask the Doc, Youth Connection (up to age 21), Other Chronic Diseases (including the Parkinson's Action Network), Travel Concerns, and Impotence (private section for men only). Forum personnel have either diabetes or a related disorder or treat patients with diabetes.

go MDAFORUM ($) The MDA Forum, online home of the Muscular Dystrophy Association, Inc., brings together people with neuromuscular disease and others who care to meet, talk, share, learn, explore, and solve problems together. You'll meet members through live conferences and an active message board that includes sections on news, MDA history and activities, ALS support, research, resource directories, summer camp information, travel tips, legal issues, insurance coverage, and volunteering tips and opportunities. Separate sections are available to ask the expert, talk to kids (for teenagers and younger children), and talk to adults. In addition to covering message section topics, the libraries contain MDA publications, press releases, and telethon information, as well as documents shared by members. Tom Bush and the other sysops have a wide range of backgrounds, including personal experience living with neuromuscular disease.

go NORD ($) The National Organization for Rare Disorders (NORD) has developed the Rare Disease Database to help families and patients understand these disorders and their implications. As part of NORD's services, you can search the Rare Disease and Orphan Drug databases, read the NORD newsletter, look up common health conditions, keep abreast of AIDS news, and go directly to PaperChase ($$) for MEDLINE searches. While you can find information about NORD and a list of disorders covered in its database on the WWW (no extra cost), you don't have access to the full text of documents on these disorders and drugs as you do through NORD services on CompuServe.

Delphi

go CUSTOM 115 Will Swann offers members of the Chronic Pain Forum "a rest stop along the superhighway." The forum is relatively new compared with most medical groups, but the forum is supportive of anyone who drops by.

go CUSTOM 238 Bob Belanger hosts a forum for the victims of IBD and IBS, Crohn's disease, and colitis. The opening banner declares that "Through These Doors Pass Some of The Most Wonderful and Caring People in the World!" Members of the forum try to live up to that claim. The database includes several programs, a group picture, and data on these disorders.

go CUSTOM 255 The Diabetes Friends Action Network (DFAN) Diabetes Forum welcomes people with diabetes, their friends, and family members. You can join several regularly scheduled conferences to ask questions in real time or post messages on the active forum. Forum members also receive the DFAN Newsletter, monthly, via e-mail. You'll find useful gopher and newsgroup links, and the database includes Newsletter archives, a DFAN FAQ, and several educational files.

```
              Welcome to the Chronic Pain Forum

                        Forum Manager
                      Will Swann (WSWANN)

A rest stop along the Super Highway for Chronic Pain Sufferers. A
place to meet each other, relax, and just enjoy ourselves.


The common denominator here on our Forum is that all here have some
sort of disease or problem that causes our Chronic Pain.
               Lisa Mear (LMEAR)
               SYSOP

Chronic Pain Menu:

Conference            Poll
Internet Navigator    Usenet Discussion Groups
Forum (Messages)      Workspace
Mail                  Exit

Custom Forum 115>What do you want to do?
```

The Chronic Pain Forum is typical of health-related custom forums on Delphi.

go CUSTOM 308 You must apply to join Friends Supporting Friends, a flame-free, stress-free environment for support, friendship, caring, and sharing of information. Topics include Multiple Sclerosis/Other Neuro (including fibromyalgia), MHA, Spinal Cord Injury, Chemical Injury, Ataxia, Chronic Fatigue, Seizures, Cancer Support Group, Cardiac/BP/Vascular, Diabetes Support, Visually Impaired/Blind, Asthma/Other Respiratory, Arthritis/RA/DJD, Special Diets, General Discussion, Medical Updates/Information, Communications, and Biographies. You'll find a large database with software and informative files and Internet connections to both educational and fun spots. The forum schedules conferences on various medical topics. Your forum host is Sue Mark, who is joined by a wonderful group of cohosts.

go CUSTOM 388 Bruce Whealton hosts the Lung Disorders Forum, which addresses everything from asthma to tuberculosis and cystic fibrosis to emphysema, with related complications and disorders in between. Members share information about treatment and recent research developments, and form online pen pals with others going through similar experiences.

Prodigy

jump CROHNS The Crohn's & Colitis Foundation of America (CCFA) has established a forum on Prodigy for anyone interested in these and related conditions. You can post questions for physicians on the Ask the Specialist BB. The Progress in Research page updates advances in epidemiological and clinical research, including work in genetics and immunology. The Library offers basic facts about Crohn's disease and colitis and helps to answer questions about diagnosis, complications, medications, surgery, coping strategies, and insurance and legal issues. You'll also find a glossary, and be invited to contact the CCFA with your question (easy e-mail access on the main page of the Forum) if you don't find what you're looking for. The News Updates page reports on a variety of stories, including new treatments, opportunities for joining clinical trials, and fund-raising activities.

9
Neurologic disorders

*T*he WWW is an especially popular place for new neuroscience pages since it can display magnetic resonance and computed tomography images of neurological anatomy. The neuroscience community also has several active mailing lists and newsgroups. However, many are academic in tone and content and not very accessible to the general public.

There is some overlap of issues discussed here and in *Mental health and psychology* (chapter 10), so be sure to check both places. If you're looking for information and support for a disability caused by a brain injury or other neurologic condition, check in chapter 14. For more information on brain tumors, see chapter 7.

Alzheimer's disease
Alzheimer Society of Ottawa-Carleton
(http://www.ncf.carleton.ca/go.html, select Alzheimer),
Alzheimer Web (http://werple.mira.net.au/~dhs/ad.html),
Alzheimer (majordomo@wubios.wustl.edu),
Alzheimer's Information Center
(telnet freenet.hsc.colorado.edu, login GUEST)

For a comprehensive review of online sources of information about Alzheimer's disease, see chapter 4, *Sample search for online medical information*.

Amyotrophic lateral sclerosis (ALS)
ALS mailing list (bro@huey.met.fsu.edu)

Moderated by Bob Broedel, the ALS mailing list reaches out weekly to the global ALS community. At the end of 1994, more than 400 subscribers had joined. The list invites patients, friends and families of patients, caregivers, clinicians, researchers, and anyone else interested in ALS (also known as Lou Gehrig's disease or motor neuron disease) to join. You'll find lots of news (including wire stories), online and offline resources, patient experiences, requests for participation and help from researchers, and support. Because this list doesn't go through an automated list server, send e-mail to Bob Broedel asking to be placed on the list.

Back and spinal cord injury
Cure Paralysis Now (http://www.infowest.com/cpn/index.html),
Backs-L (listserv@moose.uvm.edul)

The Web site for Cure Paralysis Now supports professional research directed to the eventual cure of spinal cord paralysis. Participating organizations include the American Paralysis Association, Paralyzed Veterans of America, National Spinal Cord Injury Association, Spinal Cord Injury Network, Spinal Cord Society, Help Them Walk Again, and National Rehabilitation Center. At this site you'll learn about pioneers in spinal injury awareness, read true stories of spinal cord paralysis, find information about participating in a newsgroup, and receive contact information about support groups. You can also view images of the spinal column. The Backs-L discussion group, which includes both healthcare professionals and patients, discusses research on the causes, treatment, and disabilities associated with back pain.

Help is but a message away

When you have nowhere to turn to, no one to help you, and the doctors have said, "I'm sorry, but we've done all we can," people ultimately turn to each other. In 1991, I entered a whole new world . . . computer assisted learning . . . learning by talking to others rather than reading a textbook . . . the information superhighway.

The echoes are full of people helping people. When I returned from weekly visits to a pain clinic, I would create messages for the Chronic Pain echo and the Spinal Injury echo describing what was said. I would type in and upload the hand-outs I was given and explain what the doctor had said to me or tried to do for me. I did this because I felt this was something I could do to contribute. If it helped even one person, I felt my life meant something. About halfway into the six-week outpatient course at the pain clinic, it was obvious that nothing they said or did was helping me lower my chronic pain. I could have given up, but I wanted to continue to help others online. Now when someone asks if there is anyone who has been to a pain clinic, I can tell them of my experiences or send them a file. What didn't help me might help someone else.

Similarly, not too many people in the U.S. have had an implanted spinal cord stimulator, but it's going to be routine in the not-too-distant future. I've had the full surgery once and a replacement battery pack once. I've told of my experiences online. I also wrote a file that explains how it's done, what the effects are, what the patient will feel, and my personal notes. Again, it makes me feel useful.

Of course, if you keep complaining, no one wants to talk to you after awhile. I try to show people that one of my ways to fight the chronic pain is with humor. This might take a few people time to understand, but it's such a joy to watch someone new come into the echo and react to me and others using humor to fight the pain. If we can't laugh at ourselves, then there is no hope. After the new people get to know everyone, they're part of our little family.

Joining in on the Internet and sharing information can be enlightening as well as humorous. You learn much, but you wind up giving so much more to others. Once you find your way through the "ins and outs" of BBSing, I'm sure you'll agree that this is one of the best ways to be in touch with people. See you on the echoes!

Linda Cummings
Mobile, Ala.

Brain injury

bit.listserv.tbi-support, TBI-Sprt (listserv@sjuvm.stjohns.edu),
Traumatic Brain Injury (gopher:// gopher.sasquatch.com:70 or
http://www.sasquatch.com/tbi)

The TBI-Sprt mailing list promotes the exchange of information among survivors, supporters, and professionals concerned with traumatic brain injury and other neurological impairments that currently lack a forum. You can receive information from this list by subscribing to the mailing list or the digest version, to the list's index (and ordering individual messages), or to the moderated bit.listserv.tbi-support newsgroup. You'll also find the mailing list on various gophers and Web sites, including the St. John's University gopher and Web pages. Like all St. John's University mailing lists, TBI-Sprt is well-maintained and full of useful information, resources, and support.

Len Burns, owner of TBI-Sprt, has also established the Sasquatch Gopher Server with considerable help from Dena Taylor, executive director of The Perspectives Network (TPN). You'll find a description of TPN and the services it provides, the TPN FAQ, the TPN resources list, electronic editions of *TPN* magazine, articles from the TBI-Sprt file list, archives of the more substantial

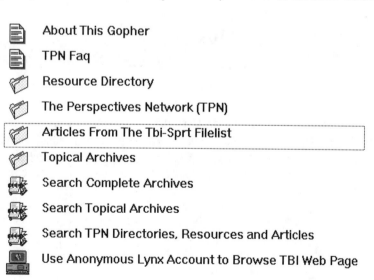

The TBI gopher covers traumatic brain injuries.

TBI-Sprt discussion threads (sorted by topic and date), various searching tools (by keyword of document text), and a telnet connection (using Lynx) to the Web site that provides the same archives and searching capabilities.

Cerebral palsy

alt.support.cerebral-palsy, C-Palsy (listserv@sjuvm.stjohns.edu),
Our-Kids (our-kids-request@tbag.osc.edu),
Our-Kids Home Page (http://wonder.mit.edu/our-kids.html)

People with cerebral palsy, their supporters and caregivers, physicians, and researchers are among C-Palsy mailing list subscribers. The list encourages members to share personal experiences and discuss treatment issues. You can also join the CPalsy conference on Fidonet or the less active Usenet newsgroup.

Parents of children with cerebral palsy should read Our-Kids or visit the sophisticated Our-Kids Web pages. Available are archives of the list, nutrition tips, links to the Arc and ABLEDATA (chapter 14, *Disabilities*), and information about and links to sites on autism, cerebral palsy, and Down's syndrome.

Dystonia

alt.support.dystonia

Patients dealing with dystonia, both a symptom and the name for a group of illnesses, can turn to alt.support dystonia for information, support, and discussion. Trudy Mason offers a concise Dystonia FAQ, which includes details for contacting the Dystonia Medical Research Foundation. This small discussion group shares experiences about specific types of dystonia and reaches out to anyone seeking help.

Epilepsy

alt.support.epilepsy, Epilepsy-List (listserv@calvin.dgbt.doc.ca),
Epilepsy Page (http://www.swcp.com/~djf/epilepsy/),
Conversational Hypertext Access Technology
(telnet debra.dgbt.doc.ca 3000)

For discussions about epilepsy and seizure disorders, you can join either the Usenet newsgroup alt.support.epilepsy or the Epilepsy-List mailing list. Participants include epilepsy patients, their friends and relatives, healthcare professionals, and researchers. At both sites you can discuss symptoms, drugs, miscellaneous topics (such as surgery and dental care), and the latest epilepsy news. You'll also find members posting general information about epilepsy, including glossaries of epilepsy terms and explanations of how to handle a person having a seizure.

Another way to learn more about epilepsy is to telnet to CHAT, an information retrieval technology that allows you to ask questions in normal English sentences and get answers from the very responsive CHAT system (see chapter 6 for instructions on using CHAT).

With help from contributors, Dale J. Frederick has started an Epilepsy Web page that provides text, graphic files, and links to related resources. You can jump from the top index to What's New, Epilepsy Specific, Neuroscience and Neurobiology, Pharmaceutical Information, and Disability Resources. You can also read a summary of epilepsy, find out how to contact the Epilepsy Foundation of America, check reviews of books on the condition, telnet to the Washington University Medical Library Epilepsy Database and CHAT, view a brain scan of a seizure, and read about new theories and treatments.

Headache

alt.support.headaches.migraines, Headache (listserv@shsu.edu)

Initiated by Leonard Zimmermann, the alt.support.headaches.migraines newsgroup offers a forum for discussing the prevention, treatment, and coping strategies for migraine, cluster, and other severe headaches. Common topics include current and new drugs, headache triggers, and dietary suggestions. The active group also maintains a comprehensive FAQ.

For more general discussion about many types of headaches including migraine, cluster and vascular, join the Headache mailing list. There you can share your experiences about headache treatments, seasonal changes in symptoms, strategies for traveling, and headache triggers, such as specific foods.

Multiple sclerosis
alt.support.mult-sclerosis, MSlist-L (listserv@technion.technion.ac.il),
Multiple Sclerosis Information (http://www.infosci.org/)

If you have questions about multiple sclerosis and want answers from patients and healthcare professionals, the alt.support.mult-sclerosis newsgroup is a good place to start. Here you'll find postings of both the MS FAQ and the Fidonet Multi_Sclerosis conference. You can also exchange postings with Dr. Chanoch Weil's MSlist-L. No matter which group you join, you can share information, experiences, and support on a wide range of topics related to the disease and its treatment, including specific clinics, drugs, and homeopathic remedies. You'll learn about offline sources of information and discussion of issues related to the Americans with Disabilities Act. Members often post announcements of new clinical trials and can help you learn more about a particular trial if you ask.

If you can access the Web, make your first stop at INFOSCI's Home Page. This Web site, maintained by the U.K. Multiple Sclerosis Society, contains many text and HTML documents of interest, including physician-authored articles on bladder function, bowel problems, cognitive and perceptual problems, exercise, and other challenges associated with MS. You'll also find many documents written from a patient's perspective, including articles about dealing with fatigue, stress, anger, sexual dysfunction, and even playing the violin. Other articles discuss current and experimental treatments for multiple sclerosis.

You'll also find FAQs for the alt.support.mult-sclerosis newsgroup and MSlist, and a two-part FAQ on the Swank diet. The articles are written in several languages (including English). You'll find links to other online resources related to

MS, such as The Whole Brain Atlas (see the entry later in this chapter), which includes brain images taken over time of a patient with MS.

Neuroscience guides
Neurosciences Internet Resource Guide
http://http2.sils.umich.edu/Public/nirg/nirg1.html

This extensive, up-to-date, very readable guide to Internet neuroscience resources exists both as a text document and a Web page with hypertext links. The authors, Sheryl Cormicle and Steve Bonario, prepared this guide as part of course work in the School of Information and Library Studies at the University of Michigan. Individuals with a background in biology, chemistry, medicine, engineering, radiology, pharmacology, and computer science will find the guide useful. The authors index the guide in three ways: alphabetically by resource name, by keyword, and by resource type (gopher, FTP, WWW, image library, FAQ, etc.). When you select an entry, you first get a description of the resource, including a personal evaluation by the authors. After reading what's available at the selected site, you can often go to that resource via a direct link.

– 147 –

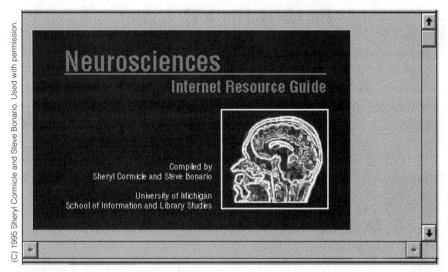

You'll find many online guides to neuroscience sites.

Neurobiology

http://golgi.harvard.edu/biopages/neuro.html

As with the University of Michigan guide, the Harvard Neurobiology index is most useful to scientists and clinicians. However, you can use both to keep up with the latest online neurologic resources or locate specific researchers or physicians. Neurobiology is maintained by Keith Robison, who runs the rest of the WWW Virtual Library. Neurobiology is updated regularly and provides access to documents and links to other resources.

Neurosciences on the Internet

http://www.lm.com/~nab

Yet another guide to online neuroscience resources, Dr. Neil Busis' catalog lists sites that are ideal starting points for in-depth exploration. This Web site will take you to other neuroscience guides, resources from academic centers, professional organizations, image databases, software collections, electronic journals, newsgroups, other related medical and biological resources, and several Web gateways and searchable indices.

Parkinson's disease

Parkinsn (listserv@vm.utcc.utoronto.ca)

If you join Barbara Patterson's Parkinsn discussion group (also known as the Parkinson's Disease Information Exchange Network), you'll receive encouragement, support, and information from individuals with Parkinson's disease, family members and friends, researchers, and physicians. You can ask questions, keep up with research advances, discuss the latest treatment, and request and offer support throughout the network. You can discuss any topic related to Parkinson's disease, including hallucinations, new drugs, research advances, and dealing with the challenges posed by the disease. At the start of 1995, this group had subscribers from 21 countries as diverse as Malaysia, Norway, Costa Rica, and Taiwan.

Spina bifida
alt.support.spina-bifida

The dedicated efforts of a few members have led to increased participation on this newsgroup. At least one Web page is probably available by now. If you're looking for support and information dealing with spina bifida, this is the place to turn.

It's easy to think of the Internet as a vast, impersonal computer network, but it's really just a very large community, like any other community you might live in or visit. Since I have spina bifida, I wanted to find some disability resources online. I did a little searching and was thrilled to find the alt.support.spina-bifida newsgroup. Every day for two months I checked in, but no one ever posted. I was very disappointed to realize no one was participating. So I left a short post, asking if anyone else was out there reading. Much to my surprise, within a week I'd received a few dozen pieces of e-mail from people who read the group. Most said that they weren't posting because "no one else did." All the others said they were too shy to send their messages publicly. I found some new Net friends, but it seemed like a real waste to leave the newsgroup empty.

If my one little post got that many responses, I knew there had to be a lot of other people who were interested in the group. So I tried to get it going. I started leaving messages and asking questions. I asked all the people who'd e-mailed me to post as well. Then I thought about what else we could do to get things going. We needed a FAQ to tell people what the group was all about, answer some of the more common questions, and direct people to other helpful resources. I also thought a spina bifida mailing list would be a great idea. Many of the people who'd written me said they were shy or were, for whatever reason, uncomfortable posting to a public newsgroup. So it seemed to me that a mailing list, in addition to the newsgroup, would get a lot of subscriptions and allow more people to participate. I like to play around on the World Wide Web, so I searched for a link to other spina bifida resources. When I didn't find any, I decided to make one myself.

After all this, alt.support.spina-bifida is alive and well. We don't have the highest traffic on Usenet, but we're doing great. Together, we created the kind of newsgroup we'd all been looking for. We have someone writing a FAQ for the group, there's already a very active mailing list, and my Web page should be up and running soon.

My point is that the Internet isn't about computers at all. It's about the people sitting at the keyboards behind them. You can find just about anything online. And if you don't find what you need, go ahead and try to make it! All you have to do is start typing. Last year I didn't know how to turn on a computer. This year I got a newsgroup up and running. You can, too. See you online!

Sabine van den Bergh
Diva, Inc.

Stroke

Stroke-L (listserv@ukcc.uky.edu),
Stroke archives (gopher://otpt-gopher.ups.edu/,
go to Occupational Therapy Physical Therapy Archives)

Bob Moore's Stroke list allows subscribers to share information, opinions, and ideas and ask questions about strokes, stroke rehabilitation, and risk factors. You'll meet stroke survivors, their friends and relatives, researchers, and other medical professionals, including, for example, the director of a large university hospital stroke unit. The list discusses the issues and experiences brought on by a stroke at any age. It also covers related topics, such as depression, adjunctive therapy, drugs, and imaging procedures. You'll appreciate the list's format, which provides a table of contents and posts the number of lines for each day's messages.

Tourette's syndrome

alt.support.tourette

This active newsgroup will keep you informed and give you support and encouragement. You'll read about various topics related to Tourette's syndrome and other tic disorders, including diagnosis, treatment, insurance issues, and daily life. You'll also find out about other online and offline support groups and sources of information. The group has prepared a FAQ that reviews Tourette's syndrome, impulses (tics and others), related disorders, treatment, living with Tourette's, national organizations, and recommended reading. On Fidonet, tag Tourettes for information and support.

Whole Brain Atlas

http://www.med.harvard.edu/AANLIB/home.html

The Whole Brain Atlas integrates clinical information with magnetic resonance (MR), computer tomography (CT), and nuclear medicine images. The atlas

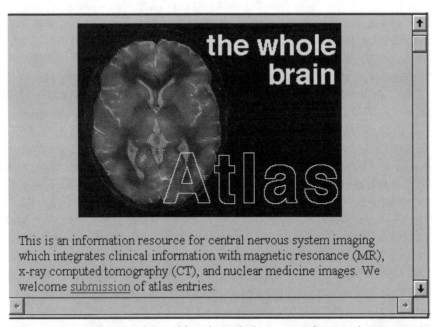

For patients and researchers alike, the Whole Brain Atlas is a fascinating place to visit.

depicts a normal brain, showing its structure, function and vascular anatomy. The site also offers case studies of anaplastic astrocytoma, stroke, Alzheimer's disease, multiple sclerosis (in time-lapse movies), chronic subdural hematoma, and Huntington's disease. The atlas covers various disorders of the central nervous system including those of vascular, inflammatory, infectious, degenerative, neoplastic, and traumatic origins.

Commercial services
America Online

keyword NMSS The National Multiple Sclerosis Society sponsors a searchable forum that provides many useful resources for people with MS, their families and friends, and clinicians and researchers in this field. You'll find pamphlets published by the Society, articles reproduced from the MS Quarterly Report, and documents from the Compendium of Multiple Sclerosis Information Database. A special section on Empowerment and MS includes practical information for the patient, the family, and anyone involved with treating MS. You can read about what MS is, who gets it, and how to recognize its symptoms as well as book reviews to help you decide where else to turn for information. The forum covers research highlights, treatments for the disease and its individual symptoms, and unorthodox therapies (acupuncture, marijuana, hyperbaric oxygen, and others). Not surprisingly, the MS message board is extremely busy. A similar but scaled-back version of this forum exists on Prodigy.

keyword UCPA The United Cerebral Palsy Associations, Inc., the leading source of information on cerebral palsy nationwide, hosts a searchable forum on AOL that offers access to software libraries, dozens of useful files, a conference room, an active message center, and resources for individuals and families. You'll find dozens of documents that the UCPA currently distributes in newsletters and publications as well as specialized materials, including basic information about cerebral palsy. You'll be updated about progress in cerebral palsy research, state and federal legislative developments, and services for individuals and families. Software libraries contain files on assistive technology, employment of individuals with disabilities, education, accessibility, and the independence and empowerment of individuals with cerebral palsy and other disabilities (including those related to AIDS, deafness, and muscular dystrophy).

Delphi

go CUSTOM 215 You must apply to join MS and Other Neuro-Related Disorders Custom Forum. This private medical support forum covers multiple sclerosis, chronic fatigue syndrome, arthritis, neuropathies, Parkinson's disease, dystrophies and atrophies, lupus, ataxia, fibromyalgia, migraine headaches, brain injury, spinal cord injury, and other disorders and disabilities. Members with these disorders and their caregivers, family members, and friends all participate. You'll find general discussions, and in a separate area you'll find answers to members' medical questions. The forum prohibits foul language and frowns on flaming. Children are welcome, particularly if they have questions about a parent or friend who's disabled. Regularly scheduled conferences give members the opportunity to get together and chat casually.

go CUSTOM 221 The Living with Brain Injury forum, hosted by The Perspectives Network, Inc. and managed by Dena K. Taylor, offers a supportive community for survivors of brain injury, their families and friends, and the professionals working with them. The forum encourages members to discuss their experiences with acquired brain injury and the challenges they face. The forum regularly announces new additions to its database.

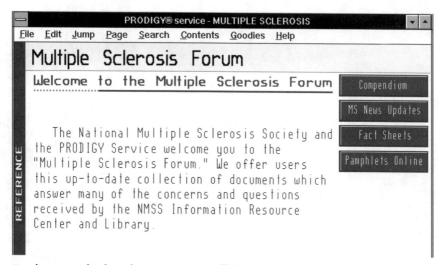

Prodigy's Multiple Sclerosis Forum will keep you up to date.

Prodigy

jump MS ($) The National Multiple Sclerosis Society draws from the Compendium of MS Information to provide a credible source of online information to patients, their families, friends, and anyone with an interest in MS. The Compendium was developed in response to questions received from more than 50,000 people annually. The Society provides fact sheets that discuss subjects such as diagnosis, pain, fatigue, genetic susceptibility, and pregnancy. News updates cover timely topics like betaseron. Online pamphlets explain the disease, research efforts, common questions, and useful resources. The National Multiple Sclerosis Society has established a similar but more expansive and dynamic forum on America Online as well.

10
Mental health and psychology

Online services are a great source of support for people struggling with mental health disorders. The Internet and commercial services offer support groups and information services for almost every psychological condition. Local BBSs and freenets also have conferences that address mental health concerns. To foster a sense of community, some BBSs cater only to people in recovery.

Because of the confidential nature of many issues related to mental health, you might want to post messages anonymously on the Internet. To request instructions on how to post anonymously, send e-mail to help@anon.penet.fi or check http://www.cs.berkeley.edu/~raph/remailer-list.html on the WWW for a list of anonymous reposting services.

The sections that follow provide an overview of many general psychology, psychiatry, and mental health resources, including information about specific disorders. You'll also find information about some mental health topics in chapter 8, *Specific diseases and disorders* and chapter 9, *Neurologic disorders*. To learn more about how to manage the challenges posed by mental health disorders, check chapter 14, *Disabilities*.

Addiction (general resources)

Addict-L (listserv@kentvm.kent.edu), alt.recovery,
HabitSmart (http://www.cts.com:80/~habtsmrt/),
Internet-Addiction-Support-Group (listserv@netcom.com),
Join Together Online (http://www.jointogether.org/jointogether.html),
Recovery (http://uts.cc.utexas.edu/~clyde/BillW/Intro.html),
Recovery Room BBS (713-242-8594)

The alt.recovery Usenet newsgroup and its branch newsgroups for Alcoholics Anonymous (AA) and Narcotics Anonymous (NA) have a long history on the Internet. You can read about alt.recovery in an enjoyable FAQ maintained by David Hawk, creator of the Usenet newsgroup. Alt.recovery encourages your questions, experiences, and advice about all types of addictions and recovery programs. The newsgroup is a good place to find news of the latest online recovery resources. Many discussions center on 12-step programs, but you'll also hear about less traditional approaches—all from people who've been there.

Our journey

I got involved with online recovery areas through a local BBS that offered them. Discovering the areas and participating in them have helped me tremendously in my recovery process. My therapist also thinks it's one of the best things I could have done. It allows me to share my struggles and triumphs as well as to read what others are going through. I'm able to share what I've learned and have been able to see how far I've advanced in my recovery process. It helps me to see that I am not alone or different.

I've noticed as well there are people who have written to me as a result of things I've shared about my own process, asking me for advice and information. I've been able to share with these people what I've learned and to offer a little hope, since several of these individuals are at the beginning of their own process.

Writing has always been an interest of mine and a tool in my own recovery process. After the time I've spent dealing with my recovery issues, I realized how much it helped me to read what others have written and to share my process with others. It was out of that thought that the Our Journey newsletter was born, along with the encouragement and support of my therapist and my friends.

The sysop of the BBS through which I access the recovery areas asked if I would be willing to upload the newsletter to the BBS and offered to upload the file to the Internet. Because I wished the newsletter to be a tool and support to as many people as possible, I agreed. This much-needed exposure also helps me receive subscriptions and donations, which is the only way I can publish it.

I also participate in chronic pain and allergy areas, which also have helped me tremendously. I ask questions, receive suggestions on how to deal with those things that I experience, and know I'm not alone.

I firmly believe online recovery areas should be used in addition to therapy, not in place of. However, for those who are unable to afford counseling, it offers a place to come and share . . . a safety valve, so to speak. I know there have been times I've discussed with my therapist the issues that have surfaced online.

Wendy Apgar
Wendy.Apgar@f1030.n105.z1.fidonet.org

HabitSmart is a Web site that serves individuals with addictive behavioral problems. Created by the California-based outpatient agency of the same name, HabitSmart is staffed by licensed psychologists and offers a wealth of theoretical, medical, and practical information. You'll find Web pages stocked with well-written documents. One article, Coping with Addiction, provides answers to many questions about drug and alcohol abuse. Another document, Moderation Training, helps people minimize the potential for negative consequences as a result of alcohol consumption. Other documents help parents deal with their children's substance abuse problems. Still others offer counsel on smoking cessation and weight control. In addition, you'll find many useful self-help files, the outline to the HabitSmart book, and The Archivist, a bimonthly newsletter that summarizes the most recent research in addictive behavior.

Join Together Online maintains a gopher server (accessible via WWW) that distributes daily news covering the prevention and treatment of substance abuse. Here you can search and read the full text of thousands of documents, including late-breaking stories from major newspapers and wire services, tobacco news from the Advocacy Institute, and summaries of substance abuse news prepared by Join Together. In addition, the Center for Alcohol and Addiction Studies at Brown University sponsors a treatment forum here that provides information about treating alcohol and substance abuse problems. Join Together Online also operates group mailing lists to promote discussion of substance abuse and strategies for dealing with it.

Several Web pages maintained by dedicated individuals supply valuable information about and links to recovery programs. Bill W. provides a set of jumping-off points for material about 12-step recovery, including AA and Overeaters Anonymous (OA). Phil W. has many AA and other recovery-related documents on his Web page, discussed in the next section, *Alcoholism*.

Addict-L discusses research and practical information related to addiction of any type: alcohol, drugs, sexual, codependency, and eating disorders, among others. Joining the discussion group are researchers, educators, and individuals recovering from addiction.

Finally, if you want a more intimate community than many Internet discussion groups can provide, dial up the Recovery Room BBS. Once you've signed on, you'll find a Reflection for the Day and sometimes even a poem or eulogy. You can write a short comment about yourself to share with other people online. The Recovery Room BBS is an enlightened, adult-only board operated for people in recovery from alcoholism or drug addiction and also for people who are HIV positive or have AIDS. The well-organized BBS offers a tutorial and plenty of online help. You can join one of 10 chat channels, leave and read messages, download files, and check to see if there's a local BBS in your area code.

Alcoholism

AA & Other Recovery Literature
(http://www.moscow.com/Resources/SelfHelp/AA/),
Al-Anon and Alateen (http://solar.rtd.utk.edu/~al-anon/),
alt.recovery.aa, Recovery Resources
(gopher://gopher.casti.com:70/11/AA)

Bill Casti maintains the Recovery Resources site, a tremendous repository for AA and other addiction recovery documents. You'll find regional AA information, the first 164 pages of *The Big Book of Alcoholics Anonymous*, the 12 steps and 12 traditions of AA, the serenity prayer, and many other copyrighted AA documents. Also available are resources from Adult Children of Alcoholics, the Hazeldon Foundation, Marijuana Anonymous, and Co-Dependents Anonymous.

On the World Wide Web, Phil W. maintains a library of AA-related literature. Documents include the foreword, Doctor's Opinion, first 179 pages, 14 of 29 stories, and appendices from the first edition of Alcoholics Anonymous; the preface, forewords, Bill's Story, transitional material, and appendices from the second edition of Alcoholics Anonymous; the AA Literature Catalog; Information on Alcoholics Anonymous; the Little Red Book (study guide to the Big Book); information and application for attending conventions; and two FAQs (alt.recovery.aa and alt.recovery).

You'll find the Al-Anon and Alateen page a good place for quick information for families and friends of alcoholics. This Web site will help you locate an Al-Anon office anywhere in the world. In addition, you'll find an overview of Al-Anon and Alateen (for younger members), a description of Al-Anon's 12-step program, and a useful questionnaire (Are You Troubled by Someone's Drinking?) to help you decide whether Al-Anon is for you. You'll also be given the option of joining the Al-Anon mailing list.

The alt.recovery.aa newsgroup, which branched from the alt.recovery group, provides help, information, and support. Members share experiences openly and give practical tips for staying sober and dealing with friends and relatives. On Fidonet, the SIP_AA and SIP_ACA (adult children of alcoholics) conferences address the 12-step program.

I had been on the Internet only a few weeks when I stumbled onto the Usenet newsgroup alt.recovery. At first I was very tentative about such a group, but the more I read, the more I found I wanted to read.

These were real people talking about real problems and real solutions. It attracted me because recovery is a very private issue for me, and, like so many people, I didn't want to go public with my problem. I just couldn't picture myself walking in to AA and baring my soul to a bunch of strangers.

The Internet provided me with a certain amount of anonymity. As a result, there were no feelings of embarrassment or shame. I could communicate my deepest fears, confusion, feelings, and questions without hesitation.

Then I discovered the IRCs, where I could talk real-time with others who were in recovery. What a blessing!

Sobriety had meant to me simply not drinking. But the caring people on the Internet showed me that it's far more. Sobriety is about a complete change of one's self—body, mind, and soul—and they showed me how to go about it.

I ate up all the information I was gathering and discovered other areas on the Internet dedicated to all kinds of recovery and all aspects of it. Slowly my little library of information started to grow.

When I first got on alt.recovery, there was very little concrete information about recovery groups (names, addresses, books, online resources, local BBSs dedicated to recovery, etc.), so I now post this information for those who are new to the Internet and recovery in hopes it will help them. People see my posts and send many e-mails inquiring for further information or just plain help.

People are desperate in their addictions, whether it be alcohol, drugs, food, relationships, etc., and they are afraid to reach out. Or they don't know where to go for help. Or they just plain don't know how to reach out. The Internet and some of the fine people who cruise it offer such help. I, for one, know of several people who have been saved from certain death and, yes, suicide as a result of the Internet.

BTW, cyberspace is referred to as soberspace by those in recovery from alcohol and drugs.

SusanB

Attention deficit disorder

alt.support.attn-deficit, ADD Archive
(http://www.seas.upenn.edu/~mengwong /add/),
ADD-Parents (majordomo@mv.mv.com),
ADDult (listserv@sjuvm.stjohns.edu)

The Usenet newsgroup alt.support.attn-deficit is one of the best places to look for information about attention deficit disorder (ADD). This newsgroup provides a forum for sharing experiences and knowledge about testing and diagnosis, treatment (including medications, coaches, alternative schools, and judo), and advocacy issues. Both adults and children will find empathetic listeners here. The ADD FAQ, maintained by Frank Kannemann, gives parents and teachers of children diagnosed with ADD an excellent overview of the disorder, its diagnosis and treatment, and how to cope with the disease. You'll also find information about adult ADD. You'll learn how and when to join IRC channel #adhd for live discussions as well.

Meng Weng Wong maintains a great Web site for the ADD archives. You'll find the Hallowell/Ratey informal criteria for ADD diagnosis, the ADD FAQ, an article from *Wired* on ADD, ADDultNews Online magazine, excerpts from *Driven to Distraction* by Drs. Hallowell and Ratey, DSM-IV Attention Deficit/Hyperactivity Disorder Criteria, and many other documents providing information, tips, and pointers to other resources.

The ADD-Parents mailing list offers a forum for parents of children with ADD and hyperactivity disorder to share information, support, experiences, and advice. Dan Diaz offers an adult ADD mailing list, ADDult. Members of ADDult discuss adult aspects of living with ADD. If you decide to subscribe, read the welcome message and participation rules.

> I grew up thinking I was the only one distracted by the smallest hum, too restless to sit through even my favorite class (math) without blurting out answers before the complete question was asked. Learning I had a hidden disability—attention deficit disorder (ADD)—helped me accept my differentness and challenged me to find others facing the same frustrations.
>
> The problem is that I'm prone to go six directions at once. Attending support group meetings required attention to get there on time and sit in a seat, and too often I shared more of my experiences and coping strategies than received suggestions from others.
>
> The new crop of online ADD-related discussion lists, newsgroups, and forums offers better solutions. I can lurk and listen to the experiences of others. When I toss out an idea for a talk or an article or ask for suggestions on how to handle a new situation, I usually get back outstanding replies. Even in my pajamas I get to meet people by reading and responding to their words and the feelings they express. The Internet provides solutions and support when I need it, how I need it, and where I need it!
>
> Contrary to my childhood fears, I find many people face the same challenges and rise above the fray with energy and unbridled enthusiasm. Many have found the Internet an outstanding tool for communicating with and supporting one another. It's fascinating, fun, and fast! It's perfect for restless, distractible types, looking for innovative ways to learn about themselves and those around them.
>
> On the road to understanding —
>
> Marcia Conner
> mconner@wavetech.com

Center for Mental Health Services
800-790-2647

The Center for Mental Health Services (CMHS) BBS supports public access to mental health information and networking of mental health services. CMHS offers a comprehensive question-and-answer document that helps you decide if and when you need help. The BBS also offers information about warning signs of mental illness and suggests places where you can go for help. Other useful information includes why you shouldn't keep your treatment a secret from family and friends, an inside look at mental health facilities, and the types of training various health professionals receive. Issues such as confidentiality, insurance and other reimbursement methods, and rehabilitation services are also addressed. You'll find resource lists for locating mental healthcare professionals, seeking help for a specific disorder, and finding self-help materials and local support groups.

Depression
alt.support.depression, alt.support.loneliness, Walkers (majordomo@ncar.ucar.edu), Walkers-In-Darkness (FTP ftp.std.com/~/pub/walkers)

– 163 –

Alt.support.depression offers active, compassionate support for those with depression. Members include those who suffer from all forms of depression, as well as people who want to learn more about these disorders. Group members share their experiences with antidepressant medications and other therapies, and also contribute poetry and book reviews. Newsgroup members regularly post the latest online resources and FAQs for specific drugs, such as Effexor and Prozac. Be on the lookout for the group's comprehensive FAQ, maintained by Cynthia Frazier with significant contributions by Dr. Ivan Goldberg. The FAQ provides a depression primer reviewing the causes of depression and treatment, including medication and electro-convulsive therapy. The FAQ also examines the association between depression and substance abuse, gives advice on finding help, and lists key online and offline resources.

Walkers-in-Darkness, maintained by David Harmon, serves people diagnosed with various depressive disorders (including seasonal affective disorder and bipolar disorders) as well as individuals who suffer panic attacks and borderline personality disorder. Although clinicians are welcome and often do participate, the group requests that no researchers use the list for study purposes. You'll find that the Walkers group has a diverse membership in terms of age, education level, gender, sexual orientation, race, and geographic location, with members from the United States, England, South Africa, and Finland, among others. You can post anonymously, and the messages aren't archived.

I started reading alt.support.depression a few weeks before my first visit to a psychiatrist. For most of my adult life I had suspected that there was more to my mood swings than just being selfish and childish, which is the explanation my family had given me. When things reached a crisis point in late 1994, I found myself confronted with a new facet of life— clinical depression, and all that goes with it.

When my husband, Joe, held my hand as I walked into a psychiatrist's office for the first time, neither he nor I knew much about how the process of healing was supposed to work. Unfortunately, we knew little more afterward. I left the office with a bottle of Zoloft and not much else. I felt uneasy taking a drug I knew almost nothing about. After a few days, I felt no better. In fact, I felt worse and experienced disturbing physical problems I was at a loss to explain. During my next visit, I told the doctor of my symptoms. He told me to take a higher dose of Zoloft. I again tried to convince myself that everything would be okay, to just follow instructions.

By reading alt.support.depression and other files that I gathered from both the Internet and a local medically related BBS, I found out that the things happening to me—nausea, dizziness, weight loss—were all part of the Zoloft experience. I felt both relieved and angered. I was relieved that my physical symptoms were normal (and when you're depressed, being normal seems like the best thing in the world), but I was angered that my doctor had never warned me of any of them. If I hadn't had my trusty computer and a modem, I would have sat in fear, never knowing the right questions to ask.

There were other things I learned from reading alt.support.depression. I read posts from people who changed doctors when they didn't feel their therapy was satisfactory. I read of reactions to various drugs and of new treatments. Having taken courage from one lady who had had problems with her doctor too, I found a new doctor who seemed more willing to help me understand my condition while treating it. Both my doctor and I found it helpful that I had a basic knowledge of depression and that I knew there were others who had sat on couches all over the world, just as I was doing, and managed to straighten out their lives.

It's a marvelous thing to have a good doctor and loving friends, but sometimes it simply isn't enough. With resources such as alt.support.depression, you can meet others who have been there and who understand on the deepest level what you're going through; and you can't place a dollar value on it.

Leigh Melton
leigh@nbi.com

Discussion groups

The Internet features access to more than 100 self-help and mental health newsgroups. New groups form regularly. To help you find the right discussion group, John Grohol regularly posts pointers on several newsgroups. In this book, we list individual newsgroups with the appropriate medical or psychological topic. Some broad psychology-related newsgroups include sci.psychology, sci.psychology.research (moderated), sci.psychology.digest (moderated), sci.cognitive, sci.med.psychobiology, alt.psychology.help, alt.support, and alt.self-improve. For psychology support on Fidonet, try tagging Public_Psych (general psychology information and discussions), Mental_Health (depression, schizophrenia, phobias, and other mental illnesses), and Stress_Mgmt (including hypnosis, self-hypnosis, and meditation).

Drug abuse

alt.support.na, Cocaine Anonymous (http://www.ca.org)

Anyone seeking help with drug abuse should join the alt.support.na newsgroup or the Fidonet conference SIP_NA. You can also check the Cocaine Anonymous (CA) Home Page, which explains the purpose and mission of CA. Here you'll find a self-test for cocaine addiction and a well-organized list of hotlines and information numbers in the United States, Canada, and England. We also refer you to the resources listed under *Addiction* earlier in this chapter.

Grief

Emotional Support Guide
(http://asa.ugl.lib.umich.edu/chdocs/support/emotion.html),
GriefNet (gopher://gopher.rivendell.org)

The first place to check for help with bereavement is the Emotional Support Guide, created at the University of Michigan School of Information and Library Sciences by Joanne Juhnke and Chris Powell. The guide describes resources for individuals experiencing physical loss, chronic or terminal illness, and bereavement. You'll find information about mailing lists, newsgroups, directories with links to related resources, and individual documents summarized and reviewed by the guide's authors. The guide is for public consumption, not for research or academic purposes.

The GriefNet gopher offers resources for dealing with death, grief, and loss. You'll find information about hospice and other caregivers as well as listings for online help. GriefNet helps individuals experiencing loss caused by death (natural, violent, or accidental), terminal illness, adoption difficulties, or disability. The gopher also provides information about the Association for Death Education and Counseling (ADEC), an organization for both professionals and non-professionals caring for persons dealing with major loss.

InterPsych

IPN (listserv@frz.psych.nemc.org), Milton's InterPsych Page
(http://www.psych.med.umich.edu/)

InterPsych is a nonprofit, voluntary organization established on the Internet to promote international collaboration to advance interdisciplinary mental health research. InterPsych offers a variety of electronic conferences via e-mail as well as real-time conferences. InterPsych has more than 7,000 members throughout the world from such disciplines as anthropology, computer science, neuroscience, pharmacology, philosophy, psychiatry, psychology, and sociology. You can go to Milton's InterPsych Page to learn about all the many resources offered by InterPsych.

InterPsych Newsletter (IPN) includes news, updates, research reports, new online resources, a calendar, announcements, job listings, letters from readers, and an index. The Newsletter's articles are well-written and comprehensive. Although many articles report on online resources, such as e-mail counseling and electronic conferencing, you'll find plenty of information relevant to your offline life as well. The Newsletter is distributed to all members of InterPsych's scholarly electronic forums, subscribers to IPN, and several Usenet newsgroups, such as sci.psychology, sci.med, alt.psychology.help, and alt.support.

Mood disorders

alt.support.depression.manic, Mood Disorders
(http://avocado.pc.helsinki.fi/~janne/mood/mood.html),
Madness (listserv@sjuvm.stjohns.edu),
Pendulum Resources (http://www.ucar.edu/pendulum/),
Pendulum (majordomo@ncar.ucar.edu)

Several mood disorder resources are available in addition to those described under *Depression*. The Pendulum Resources Web pages cover bipolar disorders, commonly known as manic depression, and have links to other Web servers, including the Mood Disorders, Obsessive-Compulsive Disorder, and PharmWeb pages. At Pendulum, there's a huge collection of resources, including telnet connections, databases, descriptions of symptoms for the manic and depressive phases of bipolar disorder, and information about conferences and organizations. You can also check on other disorders, including seasonal affective disorder, ADD, and borderline personality disorder.

The Mood Disorders page from Helsinki, Finland is another well-designed and extraordinarily helpful Web server. A fast index at the top takes you to all major resources or links offered by the server, including FAQs, Ivan, Keywords, Pendulum (Web Server), and OCD (Web server). Ivan refers to Ivan Goldberg, a psychopharmacologist who contributes regularly and generously to several mailing lists and newsgroups. Another fast index covers information on medications listed by common and generic names. You'll also find a terrific review of seasonal affective disorder, including everything from Emily Dickinson poetry to scientific and clinical data about SAD. Finally, the page keeps a current list of available online resources, including newsgroups, mailing lists, and Web sites.

The mailing list Madness provides advice and information to individuals dealing with mood disorders, voices, and visions. Another mailing list is Pendulum, devoted to people diagnosed with bipolar disorder and their supporters, including some mental health professionals.

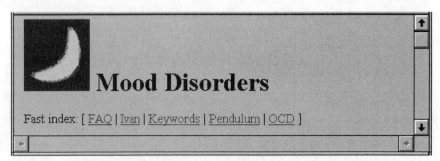

The Mood Disorders fast index will take you right where you want to go.

Obsessive-compulsive disorder

alt.support.ocd, Obsessive-Compulsive Disorder
(http://mtech.csd.uwm.edu/~fairlite/ocdtext.html),
OCD-L (listserv@vm.marist.edu)

The Obsessive-Compulsive Disorder (OCD) Web server is a tremendous resource. You'll find this dynamic page to be a source of up-to-date information on the diagnosis and management of OCD. Fact sheets, personal experiences, physician comments, medical literature abstracts, and book reviews abound. You can review pharmacological information, look at drugs' molecular structures, read press releases, and learn about many medications. The site offers discussions of personal issues, such as how to relate to a family member or friend who has OCD or how to deal with a depressed spouse. The site adds new OCD papers regularly. You can also check the page for IRC schedules for real-time discussions of OCD. And you can read and leave messages on the OCD Server's Bulletin Board Area. Links are available to the Mood Disorders and Pendulum (Bipolar) Web servers as well.

Panic disorder

alt.support.anxiety-panic, Panic (Panic-Request@gnu.ai.mit.edu)

Anyone suffering from a panic disorder, anxiety attacks, or phobias will find help and camaraderie online. The Usenet newsgroup provides information, support, and online and offline resources. Topics include memory loss and panic disorders, ongoing research, support for various phobias, techniques for monitoring and diagnosing anxiety and panic disorders, and use of medications and other therapies for treating panic attacks. The group maintains a Panic Disorder FAQ as well. In the Panic discussion group, you'll meet people who have had similar experiences and are willing to share their knowledge.

Personality

alt.psychology.personality, alt.support.personality,
alt.support.dissociation, Personality archives
(http://sunsite.unc.edu/personality/)

Alt.psychology.personality focuses on normal (in contrast to abnormal) personality types and typing systems. Before you jump in, get your acronym glossary to help you decipher terms like ENFP, ENTP, INFJ, INFP, INTJ, and INTP, which are personality types in the Myers-Briggs system. The group posts e-mail lists devoted to 16 individual personality types. You can read about these types in well-written profiles featuring famous nonfictional and fictional characters. You'll find all the information accessible and the personal stories compelling.

The alt.psychology.personality Web page offers a FAQ that includes an explanation of and an opportunity to take the Keirsey Temperament Sorter, a personality type profiles directory. The Web page also offers information about and archives for Furgis Duniho's DDLI program and the archives for the alt.psychology.personality newsgroup. You can download text files using FTP in both PKZip and UNIX compression formats.

For support in dealing with personality disorders, check out the alt.support.personality newsgroup. The alt.support.dissociation group also provides support for people with multiple personality disorder as well as borderline personality disorder.

PREVline

301-770-0850, telnet ncadi.health.org,
gopher://gopher.health.org, http://www.health.org

PREVline (short for *prevention online*) is an electronic communication system dedicated to exchanging knowledge and developing policies concerning new developments in the fields of alcohol, tobacco, and other drug use and abuse. You can reach PREVline via the Internet or a direct modem connection. Once there, you can join a live conference (more than 250 channels available), look through the Violence Forum (including the Violence Prevention Resource Collection and access to national experts in the field), download more than 800 full-text files (cartoons, artwork, statistics, government reports, research findings, press announcements, speeches, and grant information), read or send private e-mail, and read or download the entire catalog of National Clearinghouse for Alcohol and Drug Information materials. Other features include an online library of research data, scientific studies, and alcohol, tobacco, and other drug prevention information (searchable by keyword). You'll also have access to information specialists who can answer your questions. The BBS menus are easy to follow, and help is always available.

For those interested in psychiatry, the newsgroups are extremely interesting but sometimes bewildering and rather chaotic places. There are support groups for depression and anxiety, and scientific groups on subjects like psychobiology. No discernible organization exists, and perhaps this anarchy is the beauty of the whole thing. Gopher sites offer more evidence of an organizing intelligence, but it's the World Wide Web that offers a glimpse of what might be in store.

In late 1994, a search of the Web would find few resources for psychiatry or psychology. The search would yield a few pages describing far-flung university departments and their personnel, but it was difficult to find information that was fun or interesting. I had felt for some time that there was a niche for an electronic journal of psychiatry, with the prospects of no printing or distribution costs and yet a potentially huge readership. After describing the idea to others (hoping that they would do something), I decided I would try and get a few pages on the Web to start the journal off, refining the concept as I went.

The journal, Psychiatry On-Line, is now up and running and attracts a daily stream of letters. In March of 1995, it had 26,000 accesses. I hope it will grow further still, because there's a need for a forum to publish scientific papers and theories and to also offer news and support to anybody who stumbles across it on the Web. This free access is most important because I feel that doctors and patients need to hold an informed dialog about all illness—mental illness in particular. Such a dialog might help to prevent the ethical mistakes that have dogged psychiatry and medicine through the years.

Dr. Ben Green, M.B., Ch.B., M.R.C.Psych.
ad88@cityscape.co.uk

– 171 –

Psychiatry On-Line

http://www.cityscape.co.uk/users/ad88/psych.htm

Dr. Ben Green directs and edits Psychiatry On-Line, The International Journal of Psychiatry, which is published electronically by Priory Education Ltd. Updated monthly, this Web site offers a forum for reading scientific papers, exchanging ideas, and receiving advice. Long and comprehensive articles cover a wide spectrum of psychiatric subjects. Psychiatry On-Line also provides an impressive array of links to other psychiatry and psychology resources. It's growing rapidly and should be one of your first stops both for reading and research.

Resource lists

The Cambridge CyberCafe
(http://www.gold.net/users/ck51/www/psychology.html),
Inter-Links Psychological Resources
(http://www.nova.edu/Inter-Links health/psy/psy.html),
Psychology, Psychiatry, and Mental Health
(gopher://jennie.tsl.texas.gov/11/.dir/sjmental.dir)

One stop on the Web should be Daniel Sturdy's Cambridge CyberCafe (CB1 Psychology Page). You'll find John Grohol's Psychology Web Pointer, which is updated every few weeks and includes only the best links. You won't find a laundry list of resources, but you won't run into any dead ends either.

The Texas State Electronic Library's Psychology, Psychiatry, and Mental Health list offers a wide array of links to academic-, clinical-, and public-oriented sites. You'll find links to the American Psychological Society; GriefNet; and the Children, Youth, and Family Consortium Clearinghouse, among others. You'll also be able to read files and learn how to subscribe to electronic journals.

Inter-Links at Nova Southeastern University consolidates some of the best psychology-related Internet resources into a handful of choices. Some are links to other lists, such as Neurosciences on the Internet; the Psychology, Psychiatry, and Mental Health list; the Yahoo collection of self-help resources; and the

PSYCGRAD Project in Ottawa. You can also transfer to a collection of psychological screening summaries (for spotting dementia, abnormal bereavement, depression, and other problems) and two Usenet newsgroup lists, one for psychology and the other for groups offering support. Finally, you can check a list of psychology-related mailing lists generated weekly by Dartmouth College. You'll be able to read a short paragraph describing the membership, discussion topics, and details for subscribing for each discussion group.

With the comprehensive resource lists of psychology, medical, and support groups I've assembled and kept updated on the Internet, I often receive e-mail from individuals seeking a lot more than just a point in the right direction. Often people involved in medical or psychological treatment ask me specific questions about their disorders. I'm very supportive of these individuals and encourage them to find appropriate resources to help them understand their disorders and get better help for themselves. I also became an active patient advocate on the Internet, reading and posting messages to many newsgroups, trying to improve the image of mental health in general and addressing specific patient issues.

I've found that patients best integrate online information into their therapy by presenting it as they would any outside information. For instance, often therapy patients I see in the real world participate in a community support group. They sometimes bring an anecdote from their support group into their therapy with me, or some other information from that group that they feel relates to them. We discuss the information and see how best to integrate it (if at all) into the therapy. Even if the information isn't useful in every instance, I welcome patients' efforts to seek information to help themselves. This shows me, as a therapist, that the patient is working toward change. Clinicians should take a supportive approach to patients who are learning about their disorder.

I'm often asked how I became involved in online support and psychology. While in graduate school, my best friend, who lived 1,500 miles away, unexpectedly made the decision to commit suicide without warning any family or friends. He did this after the devastating loss of a romantic relationship. Nobody knew how hard he was taking it at the time, nor did I even suspect it. I made a very personal decision then to try to better educate and reach as many people as possible with information pertaining to depression and mental health. The Internet has been an invaluable tool in my efforts to ensure that others don't suffer a similar needless and preventable loss.

Most clinicians and researchers in the field who are online enjoy reading and contributing to professional mailing lists in psychiatry, psychopharmacology, clinical psychology, and related fields (such as the InterPsych group of mailing lists). The Internet is a very useful tool to help clinicians keep up-to-date in their field and receive virtual consultations from other professionals and experts. Others, like Ivan Goldberg, M.D. and me, take a more active role in doling out generalized advice to patients seeking information on specific disorders or therapeutic interventions. Currently there is no "online therapy," although researchers have conducted experimental trials of group therapy that have proved relatively successful. There are also plans to test, on a trial basis, individual therapy on the Internet. However, these plans are moving slowly because of liability and billing issues.

John M. Grohol, M.S.
grohol@alpha.acast.nova.edu

Schizophrenia

Schizoph (listserv@vm.utcc.utoronto.ca)

The Schizophrenia Information Exchange Network's Schizoph list is an open, unmoderated, global electronic discussion of issues related to schizophrenia. Subscribers include family and friends of schizophrenia patients, researchers, healthcare providers, and support and advocacy groups. Any topic related to schizophrenia is appropriate for discussion. You'll find people talking about drug therapy, counseling, and advocacy issues. Sylvia Caras regularly posts details about the Madness list. Members use the network to make announcements and to share ideas, papers, bibliographies, resources, and personal experiences.

Self-help

*American Academy of Child and Adolescent Psychiatry
(http://www.psych.med.umich.edu/web/aacap/),
Self-Help Psychology Magazine (http://www.well.com/user/selfhelp/),
SUNY, Buffalo (gopher://wings.buffalo.du/11/student-life/ccenter),
University of Illinois, Urbana-Champaign
(gopher://gopher.uiuc.edu/11/UI/CSF/Coun/SHB)*

Full-text magazines online are rare, so you'll want to look at the well-designed and dynamic Self-Help Psychology Magazine home page. The Magazine isn't published in editions but constantly changes as new articles become available. You'll see more than 20 articles written by mental health professionals and students covering relationships, sexuality (hetero-, homo-, and bi-), sports psychology, depression, anxiety, women's and men's issues, parenting and family life, grief, eating disorders, addictive behaviors, stress, and other psychology topics. Columns include Ask Dr. Wexler, Transforming Your Relationships, film and CD reviews for parents, and psychology book reviews. You can send a letter to the editor or correspond with contributors, who usually list their e-mail addresses. You'll also find links to other psychology sites on the Web.

You might have read about the American Academy of Child and Adolescent Psychiatry's Facts for Families in *Better Homes & Gardens* or *USA Today*. These fact sheets (some available in Spanish) teach parents and families about the wide range of mental and emotional challenges faced by children, including divorce, eating disorders, sexual abuse, learning disabilities, television and real-life violence, depression, bed-wetting, teenage pregnancy, lead exposure, anxiety, suicide, and relocation. The fact sheets also address major psychiatric disorders, chronic and terminal illness, insurance coverage, medications, hospitalization, and substance abuse treatment. In addition to reading the fact sheets online, you can order printed copies.

The Counseling Center at the State University of New York (SUNY) at Buffalo offers an excellent overview of counseling for various emotional problems. Geared toward college students, online documents provide information and reassurance about the counseling process. The easy-to-read articles examine the feelings, thoughts, behaviors, and physiological changes associated with each particular condition. The authors also offer tips for prevention and intervention. You'll find files on stress; anxiety; alcohol and drugs; depression; suicide prevention; relationships; adjusting to college life; coping with death and grief; and health, diet, and body image.

At the University of Illinois, Urbana-Champaign, the Counseling Center has a series of self-help electronic brochures that provide background information on psychological problems and practical self-help tips. The documents are written primarily for a college-age audience. You'll find help dealing with addictive relationships, eating disorders, loneliness, perfectionism, depression, and procrastination. Stress management, time management, weight control, assertiveness training, and suicide prevention are also covered. Other topics include coming out (revealing your homosexuality), dealing with your parents' divorce or alcohol addiction, and surviving sexual abuse.

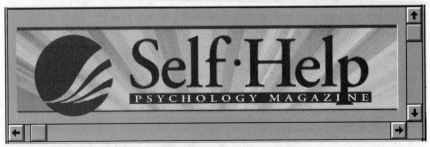

Be sure not to miss Self–Help Psychology Magazine!

Sexual abuse

alt.abuse.recovery, alt.sexual.abuse.recovery,
alt.support.abuse-partners, Recovery (recovery@wvnvm.wvnet.edu)

The Recovery mailing list is a support group for survivors of childhood sexual abuse and their friends and family. You can contribute anonymously. The emphasis is on healing and recovery through a 12-step program. The list is distributed in digest format. On Fidonet, options for discussion groups include Child_Abuse (for victims of physical, sexual, or emotional child abuse and advocates); Please (for adult victims of child abuse); and SIP_Survivor (a 12-step discussion group for survivors of abuse and incest).

Of the available Usenet newsgroups, alt.sexual.abuse.recovery (ASAR) is the primary group that supports survivors of sexual, as well as other forms of abuse. The group has a FAQ that you should read before posting anything. ASAR also maintains an IRC channel (#asar2). Another newsgroup, alt.abuse.recovery, is for survivors of all forms of abuse, while alt.support.abuse-partners is for family and friends of abuse survivors.

Shrink-Link
http://www.westnet.com/shrink

Cyberlink Consulting, Inc. offers Shrink-Link, which "helps people develop informed judgments and choices concerning human behavior." You can ask clinical psychologists and psychiatrists for general guidance or advice about a specific crisis. Résumés for the full panel are available online, as are sample queries and their responses. You can direct your question to one of eight specialty areas, such as Sex/Gender Issues, Alcohol/Drug Abuse, Family Issues, Eating Disorders, and Psychiatry/Medication. The cost for using Shrink-Link is $20 per question and response. You can expect to receive a response via e-mail within 72 hours.

Shrynk BBS
214-231-2111

The Shrynk BBS provides help for almost any mental health concern. You'll find articles, reference materials, and one-on-one conferencing with Ask The Shrynk. If you subscribe to the BBS (details online), you can ask any question you have about marital problems, parenting, substance abuse, or other psychological problems. Your questions will be answered by The Shrynk BBS advisory staff of board-certified psychiatrists, counselors, and social workers, whose biographies you can read online. You also can join a variety of Usenet discussion groups (alt.psychology.help, alt.psychology.personality, sci.psychology, tw.bbs.sci.psychology, and several other medical/health newsgroups) and chat online in public or private chat channels. Many other typical BBS services are available, including psychological, medical, and alternative medicine files that you can download.

Smoking cessation

alt.support.stop-smoking Home Page
(http://www.ncl.ac.uk/~nnpb/), NicNet
(http://www.medlib.arizona.edu.~pubhlth/tobac.htm/)

Smoking cessation is a well-covered topic on the Internet. If you've thought about quitting smoking, then consider joining alt.support.stop-smoking (A.S.S.-S.). You'll find an active group with a core of former smokers who compassionately support one another. The group tries to respond to each newcomer. Whether you've gone one hour, one day, one week, one year, or one decade without smoking, you'll receive support. The newsgroup archives particularly memorable threads and reposts them regularly. They include diaries of people quitting smoking, 10-year anniversary essays, medical overviews of smoking, and advice of every stripe. The A.S.S.-S. FAQ will answer almost any question you have about smoking cessation, including the best methods, how to prepare for quitting, how nicotine patches and nicotine gum work, and how to encourage someone to quit. The A.S.S.-S. Home Page also offers links to other smoking-cessation and health-related sites.

NicNet, the Arizona Nicotine and Tobacco Network, gives you access to stop-smoking handouts and manuals, information about tobacco advertising, tips for healthcare providers in working with patients who want to quit, information about smoking-related cancers, and health statistics about smoking. You'll also learn about several Usenet newsgroups that address smoking and smoking cessation.

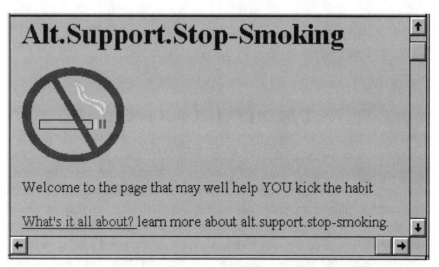

For help when you decide to quit, turn on your computer and get on the Net.

Suicide

*alt.suicide.finals, alt.suicide.holiday,
alt.support.depression, Samaritans (jo@samaritans.org,
anonymous e-mail: samaritans@anon.penet.fi)*

The Internet has played a significant role in preventing suicides. Topics for suicide-related Usenet newsgroups include suicidal thoughts, self-injury, completed suicide deaths, and suicide survival, among others. In the *Philadelphia Inquirer* (January 17, 1995), Reid Kanaley described how messages posted by suicidal individuals brought not only a flood of online support, but also offline aid from counselors and even emergency rescue personnel. Most university health information servers (see chapter 5, *General health information*) include excellent documents about recognizing suicidal behavior, dealing with suicidal feelings, and seeking help. The counseling center at SUNY in Buffalo also offers information about suicide and suicide prevention. Some freenets provide suicide prevention services as well.

If you don't want to bare your soul to the world, you can seek anonymous help through the Internet. The Samaritans, a nonreligious 40-year-old counseling group based in the U.K., offers confidential suicide counseling via e-mail. All trained volunteers answer messages using the name Jo. You can request the FAQ file to learn more about how the program evolved, how anonymous e-mail works, and other services offered by the Samaritans.

Commercial services
America Online

keyword IMH Issues in Mental Health offers a forum to ask questions, attend conferences, and exchange information with fellow members and mental health professionals. Your forum leader, Arrianne, is a mental health professional experienced in crisis intervention, child advocacy, parenting, family concerns, relationships, and more. The Parenting Board, the Daily Living Board (coping in today's society), the Relationships Board, the Divorce and Separation Board, and the Teen Talk Board all offer support as well. The IMH library contains transcripts of forum discussions, prior special feature articles, and general information files pertaining to mental health. The IMH Conference Room is usually busy with participants, including everyone from ADD children to widows. Be sure to check if there's an ongoing discussion that interests you.

keyword NAMI The National Alliance for the Mentally Ill knows that, for many, the stigma attached to mental illness is as painful as the symptoms. NAMI works hard not only to further research efforts but also to increase public awareness about mental illness. Attention deficit hyperactivity, substance abuse, mood disorders, obsessive-compulsive disorder, panic disorder, schizophrenia, and tardive dyskinesia are just a few of the disorders addressed at this forum. You'll find software libraries, book reviews, medication fact sheets, research updates, and a very active and supportive message board. Members discuss the full spectrum of mental illness, including diagnosis, treatment, and societal attitudes.

CompuServe

go ADD ($) The Attention Deficit Disorder (ADD) Forum is a gathering place for parents of children with ADD, adults with ADD, spouses or co-workers of people with ADD, and professionals involved with the treatment of ADD. Members come from 16 countries around the world. You'll also note that other neurobehavioral disorders are discussed here, including Tourette's syndrome and autism. In addition to social chat sessions, you can attend online conferences held in conjunction with national and regional meetings. Message sections include parenting issues, diagnosing ADD, therapy and medication, relationships and ADD, and legal issues and advocacy. You'll find separate sections to introduce yourself to forum members, make announcements, talk with other adults or children with ADD, ask physicians specific questions, and post emergency requests requiring immediate attention. The libraries offer files that match discussion topics in the message sections. Forum sysops include parents of ADD children, ADD teenagers, ADD adults, parents of children with other behavioral disorders, healthcare professionals, and ADD advocates.

go GOODHEALTH ($) The Health & Fitness Forum maintains a message section and library for mental health concerns. Members share experiences and insights on the mental health topic of their choice. You'll find a mixture of mental health professionals and nonprofessionals who frequent the forum.

go PSYCINFO ($$) Maintained by the American Psychological Association, the PsycINFO database contains citations and abstracts of articles from the psychology and behavioral sciences literature. The information is written at an academic level and covers such topics as developmental, experimental, and applied psychology, as well as communication systems, education, psychometrics, prevention, and treatment.

Delphi

go CUSTOM 032 The Codependency Support Group is a forum for the discussion of issues relating to codependency, chemical dependency, and other addictive behaviors. The goal is to help members feel safe online in order to facilitate the discussion of feelings and issues that reduce their enjoyment of life. The emphasis is on help and support.

go CUSTOM 072 The Healing Place (THP) offers a safe retreat for those who have been through any type of trauma, including childhood incest and/or sexual abuse. The purpose of the forum is to help speed healing and recovery. Mickie Ross hosts The Healing Place, where discussion includes family, fun, and general-interest topics. You'll have access to several gopher servers, newsgroups, and resource lists.

go CUSTOM 095 You must apply to join Friends of Bill, a forum for recovering alcoholics and drug addicts. You're also welcome if you're looking for general information about alcoholism or drug addiction. If you need help for family members or significant others, you're encouraged to look at the Codependency Forum (#032).

go CUSTOM 142 You must apply to join this forum, which is a support group for those in, or interested in, 12-step recovery for sex or love addiction or compulsive behavior in these areas. If you aren't familiar with 12-step programs for sex or love addiction, you can take a self-administered questionnaire to help decide if this group is for you. This is a place not to meet sexual partners but rather to find help for your problems.

go CUSTOM 182 Death & Dying Online Exchange is a caring community that embraces the discussion of medical, legal, social, philosophical, religious, and personal issues related to death. Information resources include directories of funeral homes and cremation societies as well as death education material. The forum examines medical and legal definitions of death and provides information on living wills, power of attorney for healthcare, organ donor ethics, and related issues.

go CUSTOM 287 The Phobias/Anxiety Support Forum helps people with phobias, anxiety, agoraphobia, panic attacks, and related conditions. Members are in different stages of recovery and are quick to lend support to one another.

go CUSTOM 340 Bill Barshinger's Mental Health Support Forum serves those who suffer from mental illness or who have family members who do. While the emphasis is on support and learning, health professionals are also encouraged to participate. Topics include attention deficit disorder, treatment/medications, schizophrenia, paranoia, bipolar disorders, personality disorders, and coping skills.

go CUSTOM 351 You must apply to join the Depression Support Group. This selection process helps to provide a supportive environment so members can feel more free to discuss their feelings. The group encourages friends and family members of individuals struggling with depression to join so all can receive support and help.

go CUSTOM 355 This forum is devoted to helping people with multiple personality disorder, their family members and loved ones, or anyone who has an interest in the problem. Members support one another to help deal with past abuse and ensure that members aren't alone. Kaitlyn Weathersby hosts the forum and uses her own personal experiences to provide a safe haven for sharing and learning.

e•World

shortcut MG The Mind Garden is a learning module that asks you five questions: who are you? (self-discovery), how are you? (stress management and problem solving), why are you? (personal values and work), which are you? (personality type and career choice), and what's up? (message board). The goal is to help you learn more about yourself and to promote personal growth, particularly as it relates to your career. You can also read about practical health and wellness

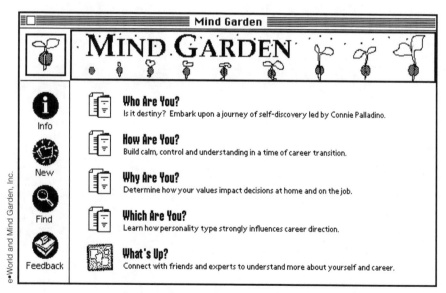

e•World's Mind Garden asks the important questions.

resources offered by Mind Garden, Inc., including pricing and ordering information. You can also contact them at the following address and number:

The Mind Garden
P.O. Box 60669
Palo Alto, CA 94306
415-424-8493

***shortcut* TRANSFORMATIONS** Transformations covers 12-step groups and mental health concerns, as well as many physical disorders. You can also join online workshops, classes, and support group meetings. Turn to Beginning the Journey for information about self-help resources, national help lines, 12-step groups, and other mental health concerns. You'll find longer files in the Idea Exchange on various mental health topics, including obsessive-compulsive disorder, post-traumatic stress syndrome, panic disorder, phobias, depression, schizophrenia, codependency, drug abuse, alcohol abuse, and other addictions. You'll also find relapse and suicide prevention tips, lists of online and offline resources, suggestions for choosing a psychiatrist, and discussion of other practical matters.

11
From teeth to toes

This chapter covers other healthcare fields for which you might seek advice and information. As usual, you might also want to check the patient education materials found at many university health centers described in chapter 5, *General health information*. For information on many other medical specialties, you can check our appendix for online resources geared to healthcare professionals.

Dentistry

Dentistry Gopher Menu
(gopher://linux2.mic.ki.se:70+/11/Biomed/
Dentist), Dentistry Homepage
(http://www.pitt.edu/~cbw/dental.html), Dentistry On Line
(http://www.cityscape.co.uk/users/ad88/dent.htm),
General Dentistry (http://www.iquest.net/dentistry/),
Internet Dentistry Resources Home Page
(http://indy.radiology.uiowa.edu/Dentistry/sites.html),
sci.med.dentistry(http://father.upenn.edu/~walter/)

Of all the dentistry resources, the Usenet newsgroup sci.med.dentistry, at the University of PA, is the best place to start looking for answers to your dental questions. Without viewing your x-rays and reviewing your records, no dentist can offer a truly accurate second opinion, but online respondents can tell you about the standard of care and lead you to other informed sources. In addition to dentists helping patients, sci.med.dentistry offers an opportunity for patients to support one another and for dentists, endodontists, and periodontists to network.

On the WWW, check The Internet Dentistry Resources Home Page maintained by Janice Quinn of the University of Iowa College of Dentistry. This Web page provides dozens of links to dental resources around the world. Many links will take you to academic servers at various schools of dentistry, but others will answer dental and periodontal questions in simple terms. At this Web site you'll also find the archives of the sci.med.dentistry newsgroup, information on forensic dentistry, and documents on the debate over whether amalgam fillings cause health problems.

The Dentistry Homepage from the University of Pittsburgh is similar in name and function to the Iowa Web site. The Pittsburgh page offers links to about a dozen Web and gopher sites from university dental schools around the world, as well as links to sources of information on periodontal disease, nutrition and dental health, and a National Institutes of Health (NIH) conference report on the effects of dental restorative materials.

One site that will point you to some of the best sources of dental information worldwide is the Dentistry Gopher Menu maintained by Lund University in Sweden. The gopher offers links to Columbia Presbyterian Medical Center, the Harvard School of Dental Medicine, Healthline at the University of Montana, a World Health Organization report on oral health, a Danish Web page on odontogenic tumors, and the NIH conference report about dental restoratives. As with all Internet access, we recommend that you go directly to the source if possible rather than via the Swedish server.

Another top resource is the General Dentistry Web page, maintained by O. Nestor Reyes, D.D.S. Here you'll find information about periodontal disease (from healthy gums to gingivitis to various stages of periodontitis), dental cavities (small, large, abscessed), and oral hygiene. You'll also find links to many other dental locations on the Internet.

Since I started the pediatric dental thread in the sci.med.dentistry newsgroup, I've had many responses from both pediatric dentists and parents. The pediatric dentists have responded positively, and I've had mail from other pediatric dentists as far away as Argentina. Right now I believe the Internet isn't really utilized as much as it will be in the future for scientific discussion among clinical practitioners and for information searches performed by the public (parents, in this case).

My questions from parents are basically the same type I receive in my office: "My child is six and he hasn't lost his baby teeth yet . . . is this normal?" or "How do I find a good pediatric dentist?" or "At what age do I take my child to the pediatric dentist?" I send replies to the questions via e-mail. The questions I can't answer I refer to another source. As people become more aware of the resources available on the Internet, especially with the release of this guide on online medical resources, I might become inundated with questions and will have to come up with a strategy to "farm out" these types of questions to other online pediatric dentists.

Basically, I'm doing this for fun myself, and I don't want to become overburdened. I'm married and have two small boys, so my online time is after 9 P.M., when the boys are in bed. I enjoy surfing the Net in all directions, chatting, reading the news, and writing my friends. I hope that I can continue to help others share information in the dental newsgroup.

I'm very excited to be a party to the inception of this cyberspatial palace of information and am optimistic that we will all benefit from our future connections.

J. Mark Bayless, D.M.D.
JMBay@aol.com

The University of Pennsylvania School of Dental Medicine also maintains an impressive Web page, with links to general Internet resources, special medical resources (pharmacology, histology, radiology), the Virtual Hospital, biomedical journals and newsgroups, dental libraries, and dental schools and research facilities. If you've checked out the other home pages mentioned earlier, you'll recognize many of these links.

Dentistry On Line, which originates in the United Kingdom, offers peer-reviewed dentistry publications and an opportunity for dental patients to ask questions in the Patients' Query and Information Page. If you have a specific question, send e-mail to ad88@cityscape.co.uk and note QUESTION in the subject line. Dr. Rob Glenning maintains the Web page.

Environmental and occupational medicine

C+Health (listserv@iubvm.ucs.ind.iana.edu), Dan Wallach's Home Page (http://www.cs.princeton.edu/~dwallach/tifaq/), Environmental Health (gopher://gopher.health .state.ny.us/11/.consumer/.environ), Health and Computers (http://web.mit.edu:1962/tiserve.mit.edu/9000/25204), Repetitive Strain Injury Network Newsletter (majordomo@world.std.com), sci.med.occupational, Sorehand (listserv@ucsfvm.ucsf.edu), Swedish Association for the Electrically and VDT Injured (http://www.isy.liu.se/~tegen/febost.html)

If you use a computer keyboard frequently, you're at increased risk for repetitive strain injuries (RSIs), such as carpal tunnel syndrome. To find out how to prevent injury or take care of sore hands, make Dan Wallach's Home Page your first stop. Dan has adapted his already incredible Typing Injury FAQ to an HTML document to which he's added pictures of alternative keyboards and other cool stuff. The document provides links to and information about almost every online and offline RSI and adverse motion tension (AMT) resource. Dan also reviews the ergonomics of software, equipment, and furniture. At Dan Wallach's home page, you'll find a separate Keyboard FAQ that examines ergonomic keyboards and pointing devices and provides information about speech recognition products and voice control of your computer.

As you might expect from an institution known for its computer science and engineering departments, the Massachusetts Institute of Technology (MIT) provides a Web site full of information on the health effects of computing. Prepared by MIT's Computing Support Services, the Health and Computers page features poignant stories written by students describing how they developed carpal tunnel syndrome and other RSIs. You'll also find documents on wrist, hand, and eye problems and health and safety guidelines for preventing RSIs and other computer use-related injuries. Like MIT, many other institutions with large engineering and computer science departments offer information about computer-related health risks (try http://www.cs.cmu.edu:8001/afs/cs.cmu.edu/help/www/06-Miscellaneous/RSI).

The Repetitive Strain Injury Network Newsletter is a bimonthly publication for people concerned about carpal tunnel syndrome, tendinitis, and other repetitive strain injuries. The newsletter includes prevention and treatment information and a discussion of legal issues. You can find back issues of the newsletter and many other documents by using anonymous FTP to get to sunsite.unc.edu/pub/docs/typing-injury or by going to ftp://ftp.csua.berkeley.edu/pub/typing-injury/rsi-network. Be sure to read the RSI Network Newsletter FTP ReadMe, which explains how to open the various compressed files.

If you're concerned about computer use-related injuries, several mailing lists are available. The Sorehand discussion group is for people with carpal tunnel syndrome, tendinitis, and other computer use-related injuries. This is the best group to join for medical and legal information, product news, and support. Sorehand might also get a Usenet gateway since a specific newsgroup about RSI is under consideration. The C+Health discussion group shares information, experiences, concerns, and advice about the misuse and overuse of computers. Medical topics include eyestrain, headache, carpal tunnel syndrome, and other RSIs. For support with RSIs, you should also look for other local mailing lists (such as in Boston and Pittsburgh) and information on freenets and local BBSs.

Repetitive strain injury (RSI)

When I was first injured in 1991 (tendinitis in both wrists from too much typing), I did what any sensible computer geek would do. I turned to the Internet in search of information about products and what-not that could save my career. I put together a list of alternative keyboards since I was convinced the normal keyboard was part of my problem. Occasionally, I'd see other people asking for the same information that I'd already compiled (keep in mind my information was based on somebody else's earlier compilation). So I jumped onto the FAQ bandwagon, the act of making a periodic posting to Usenet newsgroups to answer frequently asked questions, and started posting information I had on a monthly basis. Since then, I've built a big FTP archive of documents and pictures relevant to anybody with RSIs. I've also recently started a World Wide Web service that everybody seems to like.

Why do I do this? Initially, I was doing all this research for my own personal problems, and it was only a small amount of additional work to share with everybody. Now, I'm mostly back to being healthy, but I continue to do it out of a sense of obligation. Whenever I feel like I might like to give up my FAQ and let somebody else deal with it, I remember the stream of thanks I get via e-mail. It seems that I answer questions that a lot of people have, and I can tell them things that a number of doctors in the real world won't. You wouldn't believe how many doctors believe RSIs aren't real injuries that cause real pain. It appears that copies of my FAQ, sometimes even a year or more out of date, are squirreled away in people's files. When somebody becomes injured, one of their friends gives them my FAQ, which then points them to all the other online resources.

Sometimes just knowing there are other people out there with the same problems as you is a really good thing. Through mailing lists like Sorehand, we can share advice and experience, a priceless service for some people. And by providing an archive of useful information, I can help people get up to speed on their injuries and teach them what questions they need to ask of their healthcare professionals. The Internet is no substitute for the care of a trained doctor, but better educated patients will demand better treatment. If I can make the lives of thousands of people less painful through a couple hours a month of my personal time, I think it's worth it.

Dan Wallach
http://www.cs.princeton.edu/~dwallach/

In addition to the keyboard, the computer monitor presents possible health hazards. The leaders in setting monitor emission standards are the Swedes. For the latest developments you can go to the Swedish Association for the Electrically and VDT Injured (FEB), which offers information on computers, cellular telephones, microwave ovens, and other sources of EMF radiation. You can read press releases, a manual that explains electrical hypersensitivity, special reports, health bulletins, and research updates. Documents are written in Swedish and English. You'll also find links to other online resources, such as EMF-Link; MIT Health and Computers; and the Powerlines, EMF, and Cancer FAQ.

For more information on environmental and occupational health, check the New York State Department of Health Gopher. This server provides several excellent files, including an introduction to toxic substances, information about electromagnetic fields, and a glossary of environmental health terms. These documents are written in simple language and will help you understand any technical documents you might find elsewhere on the Net.

Finally, the sci.med.occupational newsgroup covers a broad range of environmental health issues, such as exposure to toxic substances, lead poisoning, work site health hazards, consumer product safety, and state and federal regulations. Some RSI and other computer-related health questions are also discussed here.

Eye care

Periscope BBS (803-650-9022), sci.med.vision,
Vision Science Group (http://ucaussie.berkeley.edu/UCBSO.html)

Sci.med.vision covers a spectrum of topics, from professionally oriented discussions of eye diseases and their treatments to questions from patients about cataracts. Optometrists and ophthalmologists respond to select queries, with nonprofessionals also offering advice. The newsgroup announces new online vision resources and posts Dr. Grant Sayer's Vision FAQ, which offers a comprehensive summary of eye disorders, their treatment, and related online and offline resources.

The Vision Science Group Web page from the School of Optometry at the University of California, Berkeley offers dozens of links to academic institutions, research centers, professional organizations and societies, tutorials and FAQs, and newsgroup archives. You'll find topics ranging from optometry and optics to computer vision and neural networks. A link also exists to a FAQ from Australia on An Experience with PRK, which refers to photorefractive keratectomy, an experimental laser treatment to correct near-sightedness. Although several leads will take you to technical dead ends, the health consumer will find some useful information including, again, the Vision FAQ.

If you want more information, call the Periscope BBS, operated by Dr. Walt Mayo and sponsored by the Southern Council of Optometrists. Among the mail conferences available you'll find Optometrist (basically an Ask the Optometrist feature) and Grand_Rounds, the sci.med echo, which includes some questions about eye health and that ubiquitous Vision FAQ.

Internet resources have sights on eye care!

The eye-care profession is hitching a ride on the Internet as a means of providing better information for both the public and the profession. 1994 saw the starting of a new Usenet newsgroup—sci.med.vision—for the discussion of ophthalmology/optometry and allied fields. Personally, I've had contact with many ophthalmologists and optometrists both locally and abroad. This has enabled me to:

- Locate private optometric networks in the United States, which has resulted in an Australian group being formed to interconnect optometrists
- Contact a professional group of vision librarians to determine the latest journals and monitor progress of online access to libraries
- Provide detailed information to Internet users on eye-care problems

Some of the types of patient queries that I've consulted on have included:

- Providing details of keratoconus treatment
- Answering questions on refractive surgery and collating information on a series of patients who have undergone these procedures to serve as a useful document for other individuals considering surgery
- Discussing dry-eye problems
- Offering advice and suggestions on contact lens problems and explaining the terminology of contact lens designs

One of the most unusual and interesting anecdotes of using e-mail and the Internet was the request from a person in Japan who was seeking information on glaucoma therapy for his parents in Boston. Upon answering his questions, I was then asked for recommendations of glaucoma specialists in the Boston area—a difficult request given that I was located in Sydney, Australia. But through e-mail contacts, I was able to obtain details of specialists and relay this information to the person in Japan. Of course, the originator of the request hadn't realized that I was based on the other side of the globe. When he found out that the names and addresses of the specialists had been relayed around the world, the strength of the global network became apparent.

The exponential growth of medicine and the Internet is amazing. In the area of eye care, we've seen a lot of information now become centralized and available for many users. The newsgroup alone has provided details of associated vision lists, retinitis pigmentosa groups, Sjögren's syndrome groups, vision researchers, pediatric specialists discussion groups, and detailed information on refractive surgery. The next stage is to distribute more graphical images (for example, retinal fundus photos) of various eye conditions that will educate Internet users. The Internet can serve as an important vehicle for distributing information since therein lies the power of the information.

Dr. Grant Sayer
grants@research.canon.oz.au

Medications

*American Association of Pharmaceutical Scientists BBS
(616-329-7569), PharmInfoNet (http://pharminfo.com/),
PharmWeb (http://www.mcc.ac.uk/pharmweb/),
sci.med.pharmacy, Virtual Pharmacy (http://www.cpb.uokhsc.edu/)*

The Pharmaceutical Information Network Home Page (PharmInfoNet) is a dynamic, comprehensive source of helpful consumer information about medications. Sponsored by Pharmaceutical Information Associates, Ltd., PharmInfoNet offers pharmaceutical publications, lists of current clinical trials (including eligibility criteria and contact information), links to other pharmacy resources, and even pharmacy-related art. You'll find FAQs with FDA-approved answers about prescription drugs and a moderated archive of sci.med.pharmacy with information about patients' medication experiences. Links to pharmacy-related online resources include academic sites, pharmaceutical companies, regulatory agencies, and other pharmacy information servers such as PharmWeb. PharmInfoNet also offers a drug database cataloged by trade name.

PharmWeb, the University of Manchester (U.K.) Department of Pharmacy Web page, offers comprehensive links to other pharmacy information sources on the Internet, including academic, government, and commercial servers. PharmWeb also provides information about pharmacy-related societies and groups and continuing education opportunities. You'll find several pharmacy newsgroups, mailing lists, and databases. You'll also find articles drawn from offline sources.

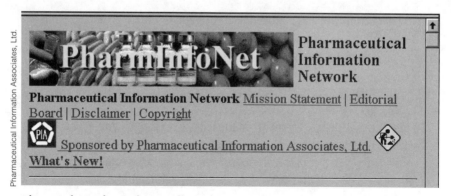

Pharmaceutical Information Associates, Ltd.

PharmInfoNet has a lot to offer patients and professionals.

Like so many other comprehensive Web pages, PharmWeb includes links to several search engines, catalogs, and indices.

You'll find a great collection of documents and links at the University of Oklahoma Health Sciences Center College of Pharmacy, which also serves as the WWW Virtual Pharmacy page. You'll note many items of interest to pharmaceutical professionals. The American Association of Pharmaceutical Scientists (AAPS) has its Web page here as well. In addition to information about the AAPS, you'll find recent excerpts from newsletters and news from the FDA, including press releases, recalls, and other medical and drug news of interest to consumers and health professionals alike.

If you don't have an Internet account, you can dial AAPSnet directly. Here you'll read AAPS bulletins and newsletters, medical newsletters, files from other medical sources, newsgroups, and mailing lists. If you've invested in pharmaceutical stock, you'll find up-to-date information on both the industry as a whole and specific companies. You'll also find news of FDA actions and drug approvals in addition to instructions on how to use the FDA's BBS (see chapter 5).

Most pharmacy mailing lists are scientific in nature, but you'll find sci.med. pharmacy and its Fidonet counterpart Pharmacy useful for learning about various medications. Pharmacists use the group to network, and consumers can ask about unusual side effects they've experienced from medications, prices at mail-order pharmacies, and strange pills they've found in their teenager-inhabited homes. You'll also find information about common addictive substances such as caffeine or nicotine, and so-called "smart" and "recreational" drugs.

Online neighborhood pharmacists

In the Pharmacy echo, there are pharmacists who can tell you about a certain medication and its side effects, and usual medical information about a drug. You can talk with others who are taking specific medications to see if they have the side effects you might be experiencing.

In this information superhighway, what does tapping into the available resources do for you? Let me give you an example. When my doctor prescribed 50-mg doses of Zoloft for me, I picked up the prescription and paid approximately $55.00 for 30 tablets. One of the pharmacists in the Pharmacy echo told me to see if I could have my doctor prescribe 100-mg tablets, which I could break in half. He said that I could reduce my cost by approximately 50 percent if this could be arranged. I asked my doctor about this, and he said he'd be glad to write me a new prescription as suggested.

It worked! Thirty tablets of 100-mg Zoloft cost $58.00—enough to last for two months instead of one. One message saved me hundreds of dollars a year!

Linda Cummings
Mobile, Ala.

Nutrition

*Arizona Health Sciences Library Nutrition Guide
(http://hinet.medlib.arizona.edu/educ/nutrition.html),
International Food Information Council (http://ificinfo.health.org/),
sci.med.nutrition, U.S. Food and Nutrition Information Center
(http://www.halusda.gov/fnic.htm/),
Vegetarian Pages (http://catless.ncl.ac.uk/Vegetarian/),
Wellnesslist (majordomo@wellnesssmart.com)*

If you want nutrition information, the best place to start looking is the Arizona Health Sciences Library Nutrition Guide. You'll find food technology newsletters, nutrition guides with dietary recommendations, legislative information, food labeling information, and cooking tips. The Nutrition Guide also provides details on several databases and other resources, as well as nutrition-related newsgroups, mailing lists, gopher servers, freenets, and libraries throughout the Internet.

The International Food Information Council (IFIC) is a not-for-profit organization devoted to providing "sound, scientific information on food safety and nutrition to journalists, health professionals, educators, government officials and consumers." Expectant mothers and older adults alike will find nutrition information tailored to their needs at this Web site. You'll find FAQs about caffeine, E. coli, and monosodium glutamate (MSG), in addition to separate directories for health professionals, educators, parents, and consumers. The Council's online pamphlets address everything from healthful eating tips for kids to food biotechnology.

The U.S. Food and Nutrition Information Center (FNIC) will give you free information or educational materials on food and human nutrition. If you don't find what you want, ask the dietitians at the Center where else to look online or offline. Send your queries to fnic@nalusda.gov. You'll also find information on food labeling, the food guide pyramid, food-borne illness, and nutrition-related electronic resources.

Many Usenet newsgroups cover food and nutrition-related topics, from MacDonald's to vegan recipes. For physiologic and medical discussions of nutrition, join sci.med.nutrition. Threads cover diverse topics including extreme vegetarianism, sports nutrition, and disease-specific dietary recommendations. Members also regularly post information about online nutrition resources and software repositories. You can find the newsgroup archive at sunsite.unc.edu. Using anonymous FTP, take the following directory path: pub/academic/medicine/alternative-healthcare/discussion-groups/newsgroups.

For warm support in your battle to lose weight, subscribe to alt.support.diet or alt.support.obesity, a moderated group. For eating disorders there's alt.support.eating-disord. If you're looking for fat acceptance, subscribe to alt.support.big-folks or soc.support.fat-acceptance. On the other hand, if you want help and support in reducing fat in your diet, join alt.food.fat-free.

If you want vegetarian recipes, try rec.food.veg. Also look here for a very comprehensive FAQ on all aspects of vegetarianism. On the Web check the Vegetarian Pages for an Internet guide to vegetarian organizations, restaurants, health food stores, recipes, and other information. Also included are FAQs from the Vegan-L mailing list and the rec.food.veg newsgroup. The Wellnesslist discusses nutrition, wellness, physical fitness, and life expectancy issues. You'll find reviews of nutrition books, healthful recipes, commentaries on new nutrition and fitness-related products, and general discussion of related topics.

Public health

American Red Cross (http://www.crossnet.org/),
Centers for Disease Control and Prevention (http://www.cdc.gov/),
International Travelers Clinic
(http://www.intmed.mcw.edu/travel.html),
Poisons Information Database (http://biomed.nus.sg/PID/)

The Centers for Disease Control and Prevention (CDC) in Atlanta maintains a Web page that provides information about its programs related to health promotion, infectious diseases, environmental health, injury prevention, immunization, occupational safety, epidemiology, and health statistics. Publications and data offered at the Web page include Emerging Infectious Diseases, Morbidity and Mortality Weekly Report, and the Hazardous SubstanceRelease/

Health Effects Database (HAZDAT). You can use the CDC FTP server to download documents you can read with Adobe Acrobat. You can also subscribe to appropriate mailing lists (instructions are on the Web page) and find links to several online sites offering resources in medicine, biology, chemistry, and public health.

The International Travelers Clinic at the Medical College of Wisconsin offers information for anybody traveling abroad. The Travel Medicine Kit and Traveling While Pregnant, both written by Gary Barnas, M.D., explain precautions to take before leaving the country. There are also a series of fact sheets on Diseases and Immunizations, including cholera, diphtheria, giardiasis, malaria, meningitis, polio, plague, rabies, and typhoid. You'll find tips on altitude sickness, auto accidents, and motion sickness. There are also Web links to several informational sites, including the U.S. State Department, University of Manitoba Travel Library, Moon Publications, GNN Travel Center, and the CIA World Factbook.

The American Red Cross, America's largest humanitarian organization, maintains a Web site that explains the Red Cross's activities. You'll find recent press releases and learn what's happening at disaster sites in the United States and around the world. You can also read more about the Red Cross's history, mission, structure, services (disaster, health, safety, and military emergency), and blood and tissue donations.

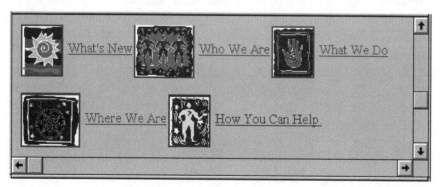

The Red Cross is online because "help can't wait."

Although located in Singapore, the Poisons Information Database provides information that can be useful anywhere in the world. The database covers poisons and natural, plant, snake, and animal toxins. You'll find electronic guides that give consumer information about poisoning; recommendations for managing natural sources of poison; and indexed lists of poisonous and hazardous substances, plants, and animals. International directories for antivenoms, toxinologists, and poison control centers are also included.

Sports medicine

bit.listserv.sportpsy,
Endurance Training Journal (http://s2.com/etj/etj.html),
Fit-L (listserv@etsuadmn.bitnet), Health/Fitness
(http://bigdipper.umd.edu/health-fitness/index.html), misc.fitness,
Training-Nutrition (http://www.dgsys.com/~trnutr/index.html),
Triathlete's Web (http://wwwiac.net/~miller/triweb.html),
Volksmarch and Walking Index (http://www.teleport.com/~walking/)

For fitness and sports medicine information, one of the first places to stop is the Endurance Training Journal. Loaded with images, the Journal covers the triathlon sports of running, swimming, and cycling (including mountain biking and road racing). The Journal offers news, announcements, and training tips, and includes a special section for women athletes. Training sections in the Journal delve into scientific issues of sports medicine, with injury and rehabilitation topics tailored to each sport. You can also learn how to exercise safely in hot and cold weather conditions and at high altitudes. The sports medicine clinic examines exercise and pregnancy, muscle soreness, lactic acid threshold and lactic acid buildup, massage, heart rate monitoring, oral contraceptives, and endurance performance. Another section covers periodization of training, while yet another reviews sports nutrition, with an emphasis on protein, carbohydrates, fats, supplements, and fluid replacement. You can check out the best clothing, shoes, and equipment for various exercise activities as well.

The Triathlete's Web, maintained by Marty Miller, is packed with fitness and training information on the triathlon sports of swimming, cycling, and running. The page offers tips on nutrition, injury prevention, and treatment, as well as

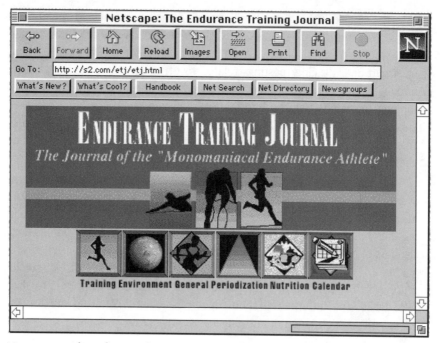

You can get fit online with resources like the Endurance Training Journal.

links to major online fitness sites. On the Web site you'll also see both the Triathlon FAQ (from rec.sport.triathlon) and the Ironman Canada FAQ.

In the extremely busy newsgroup misc.fitness, you'll read threads about body building, endurance training, sports nutrition, stretching, and body composition, among other topics. The misc.fitness FAQ is a monster document covering dozens of questions about body fat, fitness, weight training, aerobic exercise, training programs, exercise equipment, nutrition, ergonomic aids, supplements, books and magazines, and software. Created by Jeff Gleixner, the FAQ is posted on misc.fitness and available via anonymous FTP from ftp.cray.com/pub/misc.fitness. You'll also see separate FAQs on stretching, high-intensity training, and abdominal development posted regularly.

Paul Moses maintains a Training-Nutrition Web page and mailing list, primarily for both nonsteroid-using body builders who like to cook and others who care about sports nutrition. Topics include calorie counting, diet composition, meal plans, and snack suggestions. You'll also find many low-fat and high-protein recipes, with nutritional analysis generally included. While lacto-ovovegetarians are welcome, the list does favor meat and dairy consumption. The discussion group doesn't allow postings related to drugs or marketing of products. Another mailing list, FIT-L, covers wellness, exercise, and diet. For one-stop shopping of weight training information, you can go to the Health/Fitness index at the University of Maryland. You'll find two outstanding FAQs on stretching and flexibility and abdominal training, in addition to links to body-building Web sites and gopher servers.

Several resources are available for walkers, too. The Volksmarch and Walking Index provides a list of American Volkssport Association Clubs, a FAQ about volksmarching, the American Wanderer and regional volkssport publications, calendars of events in various regions of the United States, and dozens of other walking and hiking resources. You'll also learn about the Walklist discussion group, which brings together international walkers and volkssporters to share ideas, trails, and information about upcoming events. Another mailing list, PedNet, offers information of interest to pedestrians.

I received the following in my e-mail the other day (reprinted with permission):
>I have been reading misc.fitness for the last year or so and I just wanted
>to say that over the last year I have really enjoyed your posts. You have
>a clarity of expression that is so distinctive that after awhile I started
>recognizing your posts without having to see the "from" line or your
>signature. You seemed to excel at providing honest direct advice to
>newcomers without engaging in any ego-flame wars.

Since my whole point in posting to misc.fitness is to address the needs of fitness newbies, it was nice to get some positive feedback. I know how hard it is to start on the road to fitness. I know how impossible it can seem to add regular exercise to an already busy lifestyle. And I know what it is like to desperately want to be fit.

I am not an expert in wellness, fitness, or any other health-related area. However, I am very experienced in the struggle to achieve fitness and the hard body that is supposed to come with it. I am fit, but I don't have a hard body. I doubt that I ever will have a hard body. It is a terrible disappointment.

It was also an unrealistic goal for me, but I didn't know that until I struggled for years to achieve it. This is not to say that all people are unable to get that hard body. We each have different strengths and different abilities. For example, not everyone who goes to school finishes with a doctorate. While I had many role models in my life who were smart, successful, happy people who didn't have a doctorate, I didn't have any role models in the area of fitness who felt they were successful.

The only role models that I saw were the ones presented by the media: Olympic athletes, professional athletes, and models. All those people's lives depend on their being very, very fit. For the models, appearance is much more important than any health benefits. However, most people who are interested in pursuing fitness don't make their livelihood from being fit. Yet, somehow, I got the message that THE GOAL was to have a hard body.

Now I know better. I know that I simply don't want to put the effort or time into fitness that is required for that goal. I have a different profession, and I have other interests in my private life besides fitness.

I post to help other people evaluate their goals. Setting an unrealistic goal is the same as setting yourself up for failure. Fitness can add so much to your life—energy, better health, less stress. But you cannot get any of those benefits if you give up on fitness.

Jennifer, in California

Transplantation

*bit.listserv.transplant, TransWeb
(http://www.med.umich.edu:80/trans/transweb/),
Trnsplnt (listserv@wuvmd.wustl.edu)*

Started by Dan Flasar in 1993, the Trnsplnt discussion group offers information, encouragement, and advice to transplant recipients and those awaiting transplants. The group is also eager to share knowledge with anyone wanting to know more about organ and tissue donation. If you're mainly interested in reading the messages posted to Trnsplnt, then subscribe to bit.listserv.transplant. However, if you subscribe to the mailing list, you'll have greater contact with other participants.

TransWeb is the organ transplantation and donation Web page maintained by the University of Michigan Organ Transplantation Center. It serves as a comprehensive international resource for the transplantation community. You'll find United Network of Organ Sharing (UNOS) information, conferences and discussion groups, research updates, the Trnsplnt FAQ, additional answers to questions about transplantation and organ and tissue donation, support groups

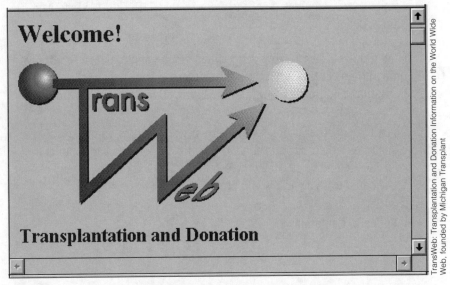

TransWeb: Transplantation and Donation Information on the World Wide Web, founded by Michigan Transplant

TransWeb answers questions and provides hope for many.

and services, recommended reading, and legislative news. There are also links to other transplant-related Web servers (such as RenalNet and U.S. Renal Data Systems), transplant centers with online capabilities, and other online medical resources.

Commercial services

Not surprisingly, all major commercial online services have information about repetitive strain injuries. These files can usually be found in disability-related areas (shortcut DISABILITY in e•World and keyword ABLE in GEnie) or computer-related areas (keyword BMUG in AOL). As always, the health and medical forums on these commercial services include special sections that deal with many of the other conditions and diseases covered in this chapter. For additional references and information, consult chapter 5, *General health information.*

CompuServe

go DRUGS The Consumer Reports Complete Drug Reference, compiled by the U.S. Pharmacopeia, contains information about the correct use of medications in general, as well as individual entries on a wide variety of drugs. You can use the drug's brand, chemical, or generic name to search the Complete Drug Reference, which includes about 700 entries. For each entry, you'll find indicated uses for the drug, allergic reactions, special dietary restrictions, instructions for storing and using the drug, interactions with other drugs, common and rare side effects, and local effects of the drug.

go HRF-4794 This Sports Medicine directory focuses on exercise, nutrition, and specific sports, including running, swimming, tennis, racquetball, aerobic dance, and scuba. Subdirectories cover many related topics, such as the physiology, risks, benefits, and energy costs of exercise. There's also information about exercise testing and training guidelines.

go VEGETARIAN ($) The Vegetarian Forum offers resources, information, and recipes about a healthy lifestyle. The many sections of this forum include Legumes/Pulses, Fruits & Vegetables, Grains & Pastas, Tofu/Tempeh/Seitan, Nutrition & Health, Vegetarian Children, and The New Vegetarian. You'll meet other vegetarians in the message section and find several useful files in the libraries (browse on the keyword CATALOG for easy searching).

e•World

shortcut LIVING WELL Within Living Well, Energy Express provides informative articles on exercise and fitness, including advice from Cher's trainer, sports nutrition, exercise and seasonal affective disorder, preventing knee injuries, seasonal exercise considerations, and the benefits of a healthful lifestyle. The Health Club is a bulletin board for discussing any health- or fitness-related topic, including body building, nutrition tracking software, body composition, cross-country skiing, walking, SlimFast diet, eye care, arthroscopic knee surgery, yoga, rock-climbing, inline skating, and home exercise equipment. Culinary Cues, another major area on Living Well, includes The Front Burner, On the Label, Eating Right Recipes, Food FYI, Quick Fix Recipes, Cooking by the Book, Wine Rack, and Refrigerator Door. Throughout Culinary Cues, you'll find nutrition information integrated with healthful recipes. How to Fight Fat Wisely offers sensible articles about healthy approaches to weight control. Elsewhere on e•World you'll find other cooking and food forums, such as The Virtual Chef's Cookery Forum, with its Cooking for Good Health.

shortcut MARTIAL ARTS The Martial Arts Forum, published by Wizard Works, offers information and research data on various martial arts. You'll find FAQs and other documents about martial arts systems, training, and conditioning. If you want to purchase martial arts merchandise, ordering information is provided online.

Prodigy

jump FOOD BB ($) When you're at the Food BB, go to the Healthy Eating subject to find help with specific ingredients, food allergies, cooking techniques, cookbook recommendations, and diet suggestions related to healthy eating.

jump KEEPING FIT Keeping Fit offers you information about determining your fitness level, preventing injuries, taking care of your mind and body, doing yoga for fitness, and helping your children become more fit. You'll also find an owner's manual for your body that covers weight, exercise, sleep requirements, skin care, dental care, eye care, medical check-ups, and sexually transmitted diseases.

jump **SELF ($)** *Self* magazine has established a Prodigy screen that allows you to read the magazine's featured article, keep track of upcoming events (including scheduled guest speakers in the Medical Auditorium), and go to the Health BB (where *Self* staffers and experts talk with Prodigy members).

2:18 A.M. This is the Internet. Countless millions of souls lie sleeping, but there are the few who cannot. Sleep eludes some of these people because they lack answers to their questions . . . questions that cannot, for whatever reason, be easily answered. That's where we come in. My name is Tabor. I maintain a Web site. [with apologies to Jack Webb and "Dragnet"]

Much has been made in the last few years about the information superhighway and the Internet. To many people, all this talk about on-ramps, cyberspace, and other such technobabble is overwhelming. In reality, the vast resources of the Net are only a few mouse clicks away. The trick is finding where all this wonderful information resides.

For the most part, people on the Net are friendly and knowledgeable. Their experience and expertise are there for the asking. There are many sites dedicated to supplying information about specific topics, while other sites are repositories for an eclectic conglomeration of information.

My Web site lists emergency service sites that can be found on the Net. It came into being one afternoon when I became severely frustrated at not being able to find what I wanted. I knew the information was out there, somewhere. One of the prime directives of the Internet is helping others, and that fits in well with emergency services (fire, police, EMS, etc.). In the four months I've been running my site, more than 5,000 people have used it to help find answers (or at least to get some good "surfing" in). I've made a lot of electronic friends from the venture and picked up a lot of good information.

The best way to get started is to get out on the Net, jump in, roll around, get dirty, and just do it. Talk to people, ask questions, answer questions that you can, participate in discussions, but mainly have fun. The information you want is there. It just might take a while to find it.

Don't hesitate to ask questions (in the appropriate places). If you don't ask, you'll never know the answers.

Dean Tabor, fndjt2@aurora.alaska.edu
Captain, Chena Goldstream Fire & Rescue, Fairbanks, Alaska
http://gilligan.uafadm.alaska.edu/www_911.htm

12
Patient groups

*I*n previous chapters, we've talked about online resources for information about various diseases and disorders. We now survey the leading online sites that provide information about broader topics, such as obstetrics and perinatal care; parenting and children's health; older adults; and women's, men's, and minority health. Since our principal focus is health, we haven't covered any of the many social, political, or advocacy groups. However, if you're interested in advocacy issues, such as father's rights, rape intervention, child abuse, or reforming long-term care, you'll find resources in cyberspace to support you.

Please remember that other online resources provide similar information. Many of the resources discussed in chapter 5, *General health information*, include sections on women's health and childhood diseases; the University of Illinois, University of Montana, and Rice University include women's health directories, as do many BBSs, such as Black Bag BBS and Health Online. The Virtual Hospital's Iowa Health Book (http://indy.radiology.uiowa.edu/Patients/Patients.html) includes information on obstetrics and gynecology as well as pediatrics and family health.

Obstetrics and perinatal resources
Atlanta Reproductive Health Centre
http://www.mindspring.com/~mperloe/index.html

Maintained by Dr. Mark Perloe, the Atlanta Reproductive Health Centre home page offers information on infertility, endometriosis, contraception, menopause, and premenstrual syndrome. You'll find an online book entitled Miracle Babies and Other Happy Endings, which addresses both the diagnosis and treatment of female and male infertility. You can view and download images of pelvic anatomy and reproductive technology, read about various fertility drugs and their association with ovarian cancer, and examine a detailed overview of endometriosis, including a form for subscribing to the endometriosis mailing list Witsendo. You'll also find information by and about Resolve, a national nonprofit consumer organization serving the needs of the infertile population and allied professionals.

Atlanta Reproductive Health Centre

Welcome to the **Atlanta Reproductive Health Centre WWW** homepage. It is my belief that properly informed, you can become an active participant in your healthcare and make better choices. It is my goal to provide you with accurate information in areas of womens health including: infertility, endometriosis, contraception, menopause, and PMS. As this WWW Homepage is a work in progress, your feedback is necessary to enable us to better meet your needs.

Dr. Mark Perloe leads the way in establishing online health centers.

Discussion groups
alt.infertility, misc.kids.pregnancy

Consult the active alt.infertility newsgroup if you have questions about male or female infertility, miscarriages, or other reproductive health concerns. Members share their infertility experiences, telling how it feels to go through a gynecologic laparoscopy or what it's like to have a vasectomy reversal. In this group you'll read about fertility drugs and their effects, both intended and adverse. In the Resolve FAQ, you'll find information about when to seek infertility treatment and how to locate a qualified physician.

The equally active misc.kids.pregnancy newsgroup will provide you with support, information, opinions, advice, and humor related to becoming pregnant, being pregnant, giving birth, and handling the first few months of parenthood. No comprehensive FAQ exists for all questions discussed by the group, but they do address birth planning, Bradley prenatal nutritional requirements, the Bradley method of natural childbirth, and many other topics of interest (see the FAQ list in appendix D of this book).

Infertility strikes at the heart of my earliest childhood dreams that someday I would have five or six children with Christmases just like in my childhood, peanut butter and jelly kisses from my beautiful babies, finger-painted pictures on the refrigerator, homemade Mother's Day cards, and shopping with the kids for a Father's Day present. One of the most basic things that I took for granted in life was that I would be able to have children of my own. My dreams were never of having money or affluence but of a loving marriage and a house full of children to share that love with. Thankfully, I have found the warm loving husband who is better than I ever dreamed, but the babies have eluded us. Fortunately, I have a strong network of support in my family and friends, and I have found an electronic support group to help myself and many couples deal with our own disappointments after seeing other women's pregnancies, baby showers, and christenings.

The Usenet support group called alt.infertility provides an anonymous outlet and a tremendous wealth of insight, experience, and encouragement from a variety of people—from those who are just beginning Assisted Reproductive Technology (ART) to people who have given up on the technology and have adopted children. Since many couples don't reveal their infertility to even the closest of friends and family, alt.infertility provides emotional support and a place to vent anger and frustration, including clever retorts to the dreaded question, "So when are you and Bob going to have kids?" Women grieve over miscarriages. Men share their humiliation over semen collection in hospital bathrooms. People listen and respond with words of encouragement and support.

The occasional post announcing a pregnancy is always answered with multitudes of well wishes and promises of prayers. These posts leave everyone with a feeling of hope that someday they will be the ones announcing happy news! On alt.infertility, jealousy is virtually nonexistent because we truly understand each other's pain and the feelings of loneliness and longing for a child. And unlike other support networks, alt.infertility gives comfort at any time of day or night!

Cindy Praisner

Midwifery
http://www.csv.warwick.ac.uk:8000/midwifery.html

Although this subpage of the Nurse WWW Service at Warwick University (U.K.) caters to midwives, it might interest potential parents as well. The page provides links with Planned Parenthood, The Home Birth Choice Web page, two nursing gopher services, the Maternal and Child Health Network (described later in this chapter), two midwifery mailing lists, and two newsgroups. There are also links to other obstetrics and gynecology resources of a more academic or research-oriented bent.

Miscarriage

http://www.Internet-is.com/
misckids/miscarriage/index.html

Women who have just suffered a miscarriage and are searching for help and emotional support and women who want information about miscarriage can turn to this very long, detailed document. You'll find sympathy and support, stories from other women who have had miscarriages, and a medical review of miscarriages written by a physician.

Obstetrics and gynecology

http://www.anes.med.umich.edu/obgyn/

The OBGYN Home Page acquaints you with the Department of Obstetrics and Gynecology at the University of Michigan Medical Center. You'll find links to other interesting Web pages, including search engines to look for more information on obstetrics, gynecology, and related women's issues. At this Web site, you can read about Caesarian sections, vulvar disease, yeast and viral infections, the nurse midwife's role in women's healthcare, and several other women's health topics. You'll also have access to Women's Health Resources on the Internet (reviewed later in the chapter). You'll find instructions on how to call the University of Michigan's telecare toll-free number for useful patient information related to obstetrics and gynecology, ranging from benefits of breast feeding to rape prevention.

– 213 –

The Internet can be a wonderful source of information on health topics, as experts in many fields have access to it. In misc.kids.pregnancy, there are labor assistants, childbirth educators, doctors, midwives, and lactation consultants dispensing information. There are also many parents giving personal experiences from past pregnancies. This mixture is great for starting discussions and many people benefit from the advice they receive, but there is also a lot of misinformation to be found.

I try to always cite references from which any advice I give comes, but sometimes it's purely my opinion—I hope I make it clear which is which! Many others, professionals included, don't do this, and often I get the impression that things even the physicians say are from their own experience rather than larger-scale studies. Not that personal experience is wrong or bad, but any one person's experience has to be more limited than a well-planned study.

People who are using the Internet for medical advice need to remember that they should consult other sources as well—books, their own physician, and MEDLINE if they have access to it. Be critical of information from the Net, ask for the source of the opinion, and maybe even see if the person giving the advice has any training in that area. In my childbirth classes, I always tell students to check everything I say against their doctor or midwife, books, and research. I give references, and I ask them to tell me if anything I say sounds wrong or contradicts something else they have heard. That way I can either find the answer or defend my position with facts. I think to be good medical consumers, we should all do this in any situation and with any source of information.

Sabrina Cuddy, M.P.H., A.A.H.C.C.

Parenting and Children's health
Children's Medical Center
http://galen.med.virginia.edu/~smb4v/cmchome.html

The University of Virginia's Children's Medical Center maintains a Web site with plenty of information and links for professionals and patients alike. Pediatricians will appreciate the clinical tutorials, image database, pharmacotherapy newsletter, practice guidelines, continuing medical education announcements, and hypertext index of childhood diseases and related issues. Families will want to go straight to the Community Outreach and Education page to view the Multimedia Tutorials for Children and Their Families. Topics include asthma, cerebral palsy, diabetes, and otitis media (middle ear infections).

Children, Youth, and Family Consortium Electronic Clearinghouse
gopher://tinman.mes.umn.edu:80/11/

The Children, Youth, and Family Consortium Electronic Clearinghouse offers links to FatherNet, newsletters, short articles, child rights issues, adoption information, resource lists, and other information related to children and family life. For practical tips, go to the Brochures, Newsletters, and Short Articles folder. There you'll find Family Life, a monthly newsletter with summaries of research articles on families; Family Childcare, a monthly newsletter on issues related to preschool-age children; Early Report, a quarterly newsletter that addresses child development and educational issues; FactFind, pamphlets that summarize research findings on children and family issues; Bringing Up Baby, a weekly question-and-answer column focusing on child rearing in the prekindergarten years; and Futurity, a monthly newsletter with current events and articles on developmental disabilities.

Discussion groups
misc.kids, misc.kids FAQ collection (http://www
.Internet-is.com/misckids/index.html), misc.kids.health

To get answers to almost any question about your child's health and development, you can turn to either misc.kids or misc.kids.health. The misc.kids group regularly posts several health-related FAQs to answer questions about pregnancy, babies, children, and families. The misc.kids.health group restricts itself to medical topics. Finally, Internet Information Systems offers the misc.kids FAQ collection on the Web. Several FAQs have already been switched from plain text to HTML, including those addressing breastfeeding, breast pumps, vaccinations, ear infections and ear tubes, infant surgery and anesthesia, and miscarriage.

Maternal & Child Health Network
gopher://mchnet.ichp.ufl.edu/1

If you're planning a family, preparing for your first child, or raising children of any age, you'll find the University of Florida's Maternal and Child Health Network (MCH-Net) an excellent place for information on physical or emotional health issues. You'll find information on support organizations, dozens of publications, and various newsletters. The gopher also includes several multicultural resources devoted to children with special needs.

Parents Helping Parents, Inc. (PHP)
408-727-7227, http://www.portal.com/~cbntmkr/php.html

Parents Helping Parents, Inc. is a family resource center for children with special needs resulting from physical, mental, or traumatic causes. The organization operates both a Web page and the LINCS Electronic Bulletin Board System (LINCS-BBS). The BBS is easy to navigate and offers access to more than 50 Usenet medical and disability newsgroups in addition to scores of useful files for downloading. The BBS offers a free online search by diagnosis, condition, service, city, state, or other criteria. Local message areas on the BBS provide a forum for discussions ranging from seizures to behavioral concerns. The Web site provides links to more than 30 pages of interest to parents, including misc.kids FAQs, Our Kids (for children with disabilities), many other childhood disability sites, special education information, and other online medical resources.

Parents helping parents goes online!

As a mother of a child who has epilepsy and developmental disabilities, I have had to learn about parenting a child with special needs. This learning about all the different kinds of seizures, medications, expected milestones, etc. never seemed to end and it still hasn't.

Early in the process, I was lonely. Now that I have my laptop and modem, I'm connected around the world with other parents who have children with similar disabilities. We can share successes, defeats, and strategies for dealing with our children's disabilities. I now work for Parents Helping Parents (PHP) at the Family Resource Center in the heart of Silicon Valley in Santa Clara, Calif. I'm a system operator for LINCS-BBS, which provides help for other parents.

After parents hear their child has a disability, we know their single most important coping mechanism is to talk with other parents who have been there. Knowing the value of this parent-to-parent contact, I often reach out via my modem and "handshake" with other parents.

As we polish our surfboards and recruit more families to join us in the waves, we're finding that those very rare syndromes aren't so rare. We also find there are other folks who share our struggle for information, appropriate treatment, and education. We are no longer alone and isolated.

trudy@php.com

PedInfo

http://www.lhl.uab.edu/pedinfo

PedInfo could serve as your one-stop shopping trip for pediatric information. You'll find dozens of excellent Web, gopher, and newsgroup links in addition to mailing list addresses and discussion summaries. Included are links to children's hospitals and departments of pediatrics, professional organizations, condition- and disease-specific information (listed alphabetically), Web and gopher sites for general health and pediatric medical information, pediatric discussion groups, and parenting Web sites. Dr. Andy Spooner, who maintains PedInfo, might have moved the resource by now, but you should find a pointer to the new address at this site (or use one of the search utilities described in chapter 15 to find PedInfo).

Virtual Children's Hospital

http://indy.radiology.uiowa.edu/
VirtualChildHosp/VCHHomePage.html

University of Iowa's Virtual Children's Hospital provides more resources for pediatric healthcare professionals than for parents, but you'll still find plenty of reasons to stop here. In the information for healthcare providers section, check out Other Internet Pediatric Health Science Resources for links to the Maternal/Child Health Network, OncoLink's pediatric oncology section, and

PEDINFO

A Pediatric Informatics WebServer

This World Wide Web server is dedicated to the dissemination of on-line information for pediatricians and others interested in child health.

Table of Contents

- Children's Hospitals and Departments of Pediatrics
- Professional Organizations
- Pediatric Subspecialties
- Condition- or Disease-specific Information
- Government and Government-related Resources
- Miscellaneous Resources
- Internet Exploration Starting Points
- Parenting Resources

Parents will find links to all the pediatric information they need in one convenient location.

RuralNet's pediatric section (which, in turn, provides even more links and online documents). The Iowa Health Book in the Virtual Children's Hospital includes information on child health issues.

Older adults
Agenet
800-989-2243

AgeNet is an electronic bulletin board and e-mail system maintained by the National Association of State Units on Aging. The interface is easy to follow and straightforward. Although AgeNet won't provide support on a personal level, you can search bibliographic databases and find key personnel to contact for information and referrals. The Information and Referral Bibliography database has descriptions and contact information for programs, papers, books, videos, and other resources.

Answers

http://www.service.com/answers/cover.html

Answers is the Web site for the *Magazine for Adult Children of Aging Parents.* The magazine covers all aspects of caring for an elderly parent, including emotional, psychological, and support needs of the caretaker. At this Web page you'll see the magazine's table of contents and featured articles from the current issue. You can also subscribe to the magazine, which you'll receive via the U.S. postal service, not e-mail. Featured articles cover topics such as long-term care insurance, personal emergency response systems and devices, and living without guilt.

World Health Net

http://world-health.net/

The World Health Net offers information and resources from several organizations working on antiaging research. The American Academy of Anti-Aging Medicine is devoted to science that optimizes the metabolic processes of life using nutrient, hormone, and drug therapies. The Academy offers several abstracts and information about aging prevention topics. The American Longevity Research Institute studies techniques designed to measure, treat, and retard the aging process. Explanations of free radical, neuroendocrine, and genetic control theories of aging are included. While you're exploring World Health Net, you can subscribe to a couple of mailing lists. World-Health-Net-L will keep you informed about the latest and most innovative therapies, while Anti-Aging-Med-L will send you current news on antiaging research. You'll also find late-breaking research news, a list of Usenet medical newsgroups, and an index of online health resources for specific diseases and medical fields.

Women's health
Barnard/Columbia Women's Handbook

gopher://gopher.cc.columbia.edu:71/11/publications/women

In this handbook, you'll find 54 well-written chapters on just about every health issue of concern to women: gynecological and reproductive health (self-care and resources), psychotherapy and mental health, body image, alcohol use, disabilities, sexuality, sexual abuse and rape, and safety and legal issues.

The articles are written to appeal to a diverse group of women from various racial, ethnic, class, and sexual orientations.

Endometriosis
Witsendo (listserv@dartcms1@dartmouth.edu)

If you're looking for treatment information and support in coping with endometriosis, look no further than Witsendo, a moderated mailing list and clearinghouse. Another source for endometriosis information is the Atlanta Reproductive Health Centre, which maintains a comprehensive file about endometriosis supplied by the Endometriosis Association.

Menopause
alt.support.menopause, Menopaus (listserv@psuhmc.maricopa.edu)

Menopaus is a diverse discussion group open to women of all ages (both heterosexual and lesbian) and other interested parties (including occasional concerned husbands). While primarily encouraging women to share personal experiences, this discussion list also welcomes the input and advice of healthcare professionals. You'll find clinical recommendations for preventing and slowing osteoporosis, suggestions for physical therapy, and debates over estrogen replacement therapy. The Usenet newsgroup for menopause is much quieter than the mailing list. You'll find the usual discussions of hormone replacement therapy, sex after menopause, symptoms related to menopause (including water retention, heart palpitations, and hot flashes), and diet and nutrition.

Women's Health Resources on the Internet
http://asa.ugl.lib.umich.edu/ chdocs/womenhealth/womens_health.html

If you want one-stop shopping for information on women's health, turn to Women's Health Resources on the Internet, written by Tricia Segal and Julie Lea. In addition to providing tips for using the Internet, this incredible guide lists general resources about physical health (specific diseases, drug and alcohol issues, medical tests, gynecological exams, nutrition, and fitness); emotional health (body image, relationships, and stress management); and sexual health (AIDS, birth control, menopause, menstruation, pregnancy, STDs, and sexuality).

Women Homepage
http://www.mit.edu:8001/people/sorokin/women/index.html

At the Women Homepage, you'll find a large and varied collection of gophers and Web documents covering women's studies and dozens of other topics of interest to women. Health-related links include the Breast Cancer Information Clearinghouse, the Midwifery Web Page, two nursing gophers, a comprehensive index of birth-related information, the VA AIDS Information Newsletter, the Barnard College's Women's Handbook, health information from the University of Illinois, and the Women's WIRE gopher health section. If you have trouble with the full address, go to http://www.mit.edu:8001; then go to student user pages and then to Jessie Stickgold-Sarah's homepage.

Men's health
FatherNet
gopher://tinman.mes.umn.edu:80/11/FatherNet

While this isn't really a men's health resource, FatherNet does help men take a more active role in their children's lives, and some health and wellness information is available. On FatherNet, you'll find research on men and children, stay-at-home fathers, and the social and economic dimensions of fatherhood. You'll read newsletters that discuss the role of fathers as caregivers.

Prostatitis
alt.support.prostate.prostatitis

This newsgroup is a great source of support, information, and assistance for men with prostatitis. Members vent frustrations, share concerns, talk about successful treatments, and offer online and offline addresses of organizations and clinics that provide additional help. John Koch has prepared a FAQ that welcomes new members to the newsgroup and provides an overview of prostatitis—what it is, what causes it, how to recognize its symptoms, and how to treat it.

Safer Sex Page
http://www.cmpharm.ucsf.edu/~troyer/safesex.html

The fully stocked Safer Sex Page will interest both hetero- and homosexual men and women. It offers articles and pamphlets about all aspects of safer sex, covering AIDS and other sexually transmitted diseases. Be forewarned that the educational materials are sexually explicit, although no pornographic material is available. You'll find a condom directory with video clips, cartoons, and text, including a multimedia project entitled Rosie the Riveter Goes to the Rubber Factory. You'll also find links to other sexuality and health-related resources, brochures on AIDS and HIV prevention, and information on oral sex. More information on birth control, new barrier technology, and other sexual and reproductive issues should be available by now.

Vasectomy FAQ
Sci.med, nwilson@actrix.gen.nz

Written by Drs. Nicholas Wilson and Michael Baker, the Vasectomy FAQ offers a comprehensive overview of vasectomies. Questions that are answered include: How effective is a vasectomy? Does a vasectomy affect male sexual activity? What about vasectomy reversal? What are the risks of complications from a vasectomy? Are there any long-term health hazards from a vasectomy? You'll find the FAQ posted on sci.med, or you can request it from Dr. Wilson.

I wanted to write a Vasectomy FAQ for the sci.med Usenet Group because, as a vasectomized doctor who has done vasectomies, I certainly feel I can contribute something on the subject. With 20 to 30 million Internet users around the world, I'm excited by the way information can now be rapidly exchanged in a fairly informal fashion. The vasectomy option is increasingly being used by couples all over the world, and I see the Internet is the ideal way to convey accurate, up-to-date, and comprehensive information to the widest possible audience.

Dr. Nick Wilson
Public Health Medicine Specialist
email: nwilson@actrix.gen.nz

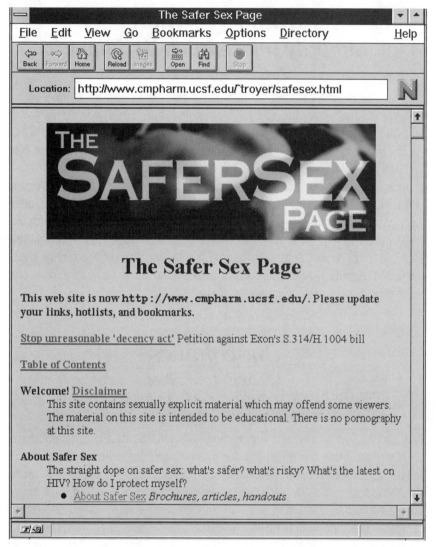

Any sexually active adult needs to know how to stay safe.

Minority health
Minority Information Exchange
800-626-6547, http://web.fie.com/

You can obtain information on minority health concerns from the Federal Information Exchange, Inc. (FEDIX). After you dial the toll-free number with your modem, you'll be connected via telnet to the FEDIX Home Page. Then you'll use Lynx, a text-based browser, to access the main directory. On the Web you can go straight to the NIH/NIAID option (and from there to minority program information). At this point, you can select information about prevention and treatment of sexually transmitted diseases (including AIDS), asthma, allergies, parasitic and fungal diseases, transplantation immunology, and tropical medicine. Many of these diseases and disorders occur at disproportionately higher rates in America's ethnic minority populations than in the general population. At this site, you can also find contact persons for various minority outreach health programs conducted through the NIH.

Chocoholics
Chocolate Lover's Page
(http://www.iia.com/chocolate/~shag/chocolate.html),
Godiva Online (http://www.godiva.com/./index.html)

Just making sure you're actually reading. If you're genetically programmed to require daily chocolate infusions for proper physiological and psychological functioning, make Dan Birchall's Chocolate Lover's Page one of your first stops. You'll find links to 20 (probably more by now) chocoholic dream spots, complete with pictures and ordering information—unfortunately, no online samples. The Choc Shop in South Africa, the Seattle Chocolate Company, Sophisticated Chocolates (NJ), Toucan Chocolates (Mass.), and The Gourmet's Guide to Chocolate Milk in the Lehigh Valley (Pa.) are just a few of the wondrous places you can go. A joint effort of Godiva and Chocolatier Magazine, Godiva Online intermingles luscious photos with recipes, trivia, and history . . . but again, no samples. :-(

Commercial services
America Online

keyword AARP If you search the AARP with the keyword Health, you'll come up with about 150 choices, so be sure to narrow your criteria. Topics include generic drugs, medicare fraud, suicide by the elderly, women's health issues, long-term care insurance, hospice care coverage, vaccinations, elder abuse, menopause, health fraud, vitamin supplements, depression, home care, assisted living, medicare premiums, and many other health-related issues of concern to older adults. You'll find most of these topics in the Health & Related Concerns folder, but you might find a keyword search faster.

keyword ELLE *Elle* magazine offers a Fitness/Health screen with feature articles available for online reading or downloading from the library. Categories include fitness and exercise (ranging from yoga and t'ai chi to fitness testing and inline skating); relaxation techniques (including reflexology, chi kung, and herbal teas); Dr. Susan Blumenthal's Health Newsletter; and health spa profiles. You can also search the Elle library and archives for topics you don't immediately see in available folders.

keyword HUMAN SEXUALITY The Human Sexuality category of the Allyn & Bacon College Online services provides educational resources and places to exchange opinions about all aspects of sexuality. This screen conveniently gives you links to Internet resources and a complete list (names and keyword location) of other AOL services and documents dealing with human sexuality. Topics include artificial insemination, Depo-Provera, genetic screening, infertility tests, menopause, Norplant, sexuality and aging, vasectomy, and gender and sexuality. You'll also find fact sheets and help tips on avoiding sexually transmitted diseases and hotlines for sexual health questions. The message center tackles everything from abortion to sex offenders.

keyword LIFETIME Lifetime Television for Women brings to AOL a screen full of contemporary health information of particular interest to women (in addition to many other features of the network). A multimedia document illustrates breast self-examination and mammograms, and a full directory is devoted to breast cancer awareness. Other women's health topics are also discussed in concert with television offerings.

keyword LONGEVITY *Longevity* has much to offer on AOL, including diet and fitness tips, beauty and cosmetic surgery recommendations, and family health topics. Downloadable files are grouped into the categories of guides, antiaging information, reader files, and conference transcripts. The Health Exchange message center puts you in direct contact with *Longevity* editors and other readers, while other bulletin boards offer more focused areas of discussion. You can also take surveys on health and well-being issues in addition to a quiz. You'll find out about the latest surgical and nonsurgical techniques that claim to take years off your appearance.

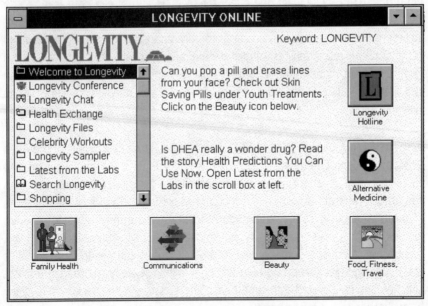

Longevity Online will help anyone of any age feel younger.

keyword PARENTING An expert panel brought together by the National Parenting Center provides advice to parents with questions about child rearing and development. In addition to being able to ask questions, you'll find health information on many topics, including pregnancy in older women, pregnancy and cigarette smoking, the pregnant father, crying, fluoride use, eating disorders, suicide awareness, healthy body image, drug and alcohol use, sexuality, and other health concerns of parents.

keyword PIN The Parent Information Network offers several health and medical-related resources for the entire family. As soon as you enter the forum, you can search its libraries, read child safety brochures, join the Parent Exchange message board, or find information on family health issues. The health information covers a wide range of common topics and is divided into folders for infants and children, men, and women. This section can almost serve as a home health encyclopedia.

keyword SENIORNET SeniorNet is a nonprofit organization for older adults interested in using computers. You can join the Health & Wellness message board to share experiences and information about many topics, including skin care, thyroid conditions, sex after 50, and physician-assisted suicide. Several threads offer support and humor to help the healing process.

keyword WOMAN'S DAY From the main Woman's Day screen, go to Your Body, Mind & Fitness, where you'll find healthful cooking tips and recipes, Health Message Center, Body & Mind Fitness, and Diet Right/Stay Fit. Articles address a wide range of topics of interest to women, including medications, middle-age health guides, mammograms, chronic fatigue syndrome, medical tests, hearing, headaches, balance, back pain, fitness, and weight control. On the Health Message Center's boards (Diet, Nutrition & Fitness, General Health, and OB/GYN), you'll find members sharing information, advice, and good feelings.

CompuServe

go FLATODAY ($) Although the Florida Today Newslink Forum has a Florida orientation, it has a lot to offer other members, especially in the fields of health and fitness. You'll find that Library #11 has many helpful articles. In the message section, there are plenty of folks interested in talking about health and fitness.

go HUMAN ($$) Howard and Martha Lewis publish the Human Sexuality Databank and Forums, a service that brings you in contact with experts in urology, gynecology, psychiatry, and many other fields of sexual medicine and therapy. The forum warns parents to keep children away from this area because of the frank sex-related information and advice. When you arrive, you can check what's new, perform a keyword search, go to the Questions and Answers Department, review a dictionary of sexual terms, or read user comments and questions. Topics include family planning, parenting, health and disease, and men's and women's sexual health concerns.

go ISSUES ($) The Issues Forum covers a wide range of topics, most not related to health. However, you will find some health-related discussions in the Women's Issues, Men's Issues, Minority Issues, and Parent Connection sections.

go RETIRE ($) The Retirement Living Forum, managed by the Setting Priorities for Retirement Years (SPRY) Foundation, invites everyone of any age to join. You'll find information about health, wellness, Medicare, Social Security, fitness, nutrition, and other topics. The forum prohibits commercial advertising, and the community atmosphere is warm and supportive. Message sections and libraries share the same name and purpose. The most interesting are Health & Medicine, Eating Right, Medicare, Caregiving, and Fitness.

go WOMEN ($) The U.S. News Women's Forum features 13 message areas, including one entitled Health. The library contains biographies of the forum's special participants, and also features On the Record, public documents related to topics under discussion in the forum. When you first arrive (either to join or as a visitor), the forum will ask you to complete a questionnaire and submit a short personal biography.

Delphi

go CUSTOM 175 You must apply to join Men Against Circumcision, which offers a place to come and share your thoughts about circumcision in a supportive atmosphere.

go CUSTOM 264 The Child Health Forum, also known as The Virtual Children's Hospital of Delphi, is open to discussion of any children's health issue. Host Arnold Solof and cohosts Tom Whalen and Lynne Axiak manage the forum. Members can discuss health issues with pediatric specialists, debate pediatric care and healthcare reform, keep abreast of pediatric news in the Peds News messages, and find support from individuals with similar family experiences. You'll also find many links to pediatric resources on the Internet, including newsgroups and gopher servers. The database includes documents, programs, and graphics.

go **GR MEN** In this popular SIG known as MensNet, manager Ron Mazur juggles several issues of concern to men, including health. MensNet has forged ties with the founder of the American Prostate Society and has press releases and articles from the Health & Wholeness Infobase. The database covers addiction recovery, vasectomy, wellness, reproductive health, emotional well-being, and spirituality. A section on Sexuality Issues focuses on sexual dysfunction, circumcision, and other topics related to sexuality and gender. You'll also be able to read the alt.support. prostate.prostatitis newsgroup while in MensNet.

go **GR SENIOR** Manager Win Morin claims that Seniors is "the coziest cottage in cyberspace." With three (possibly more by now) weekly conferences, the forum is quite lively. The database is conveniently broken into subcategories, including Health, where you'll find information about Medicare, flu shots, physical exams, and AIDS, among other topics. Members are friendly and helpful to anyone joining the forum. They'll provide help with using Delphi, online services in general, and gathering health information.

e•WORLD

shortcut **AAIN** The African-American Information Network addresses the needs and interests of Americans of African descent. This excellent forum will help African Americans network and keep abreast of news in just about every aspect of life. Discussions at the Underground Cafe are especially popular (transcripts available). You'll also find health information on such topics as psychology, sickle cell disease, and bone marrow and other tissue donation.

Prodigy

jump **AARP** As part of its online presence on Prodigy, the American Association of Retired Persons (AARP) maintains a Health section where you can "explore information and ideas about healthy living and healthcare." In addition to a link to the Health BB, you'll find sections on Health Reform (surveys and polls, state reform, AARP principles); Long Term Care (home care, private LTC insurance, assisted living, arranging LTC); Medicare/Medicaid (premiums, coverage, fraud, consumers guide, reform efforts, payment plans); and Healthy Living (insomnia, menopause, women's health, hearing loss, healthier lifestyle, health fraud).

jump **WOMEN** At this location you'll find a report on women's health and a link to the Health BB, where you can post questions about health concerns. You'll also find an explanation of the Women's Health Initiative, a $625 million, 15-year study of heart disease, osteoporosis, and breast and colon cancer in post-menopausal women. You'll be able to read about the history of the initiative, reasons for the absence of women in prior clinical trials, study objectives, and smaller related clinical trials. You'll find phone number lists for services and organizations of interest to women, both as patients and caregivers. You'll also see the results of a survey about women's health habits, including information and discussion about depression and stress, body image, satisfaction with healthcare, and lifestyle choices. Finally, there's a quiz on issues related to heart disease, osteoporosis, and breast cancer.

Women's WIRE
telnet wwire.net (login WIRENEW)

Women's WIRE (Worldwide Information Resource & Exchange) is a new computer network serving the information and networking needs of women. It offers a central source for the latest women's news and information, drawing its content from the media, newswires, women's organizations, government sources, and most importantly from its subscribers. The service also offers Internet e-mail, mailing lists, UPI newswires, and Usenet newsgroups. To subscribe to Women's WIRE, you must pay a monthly fee in addition to hourly charges for online time. Call the service for the latest rates. To receive a free starter kit including a graphical interface, call or send e-mail to subscribe@ wire.net.

13
Alternative medicine

Americans are increasingly turning to alternative medicine for treatment of their physical and emotional problems. Alternative medicine refers to many different therapies, including acupuncture and acupressure, biofeedback, chiropractic, homeopathy, hypnosis, massage, meditation, naturopathic medicine, spiritual healing, and yoga. The resources listed in this chapter and the pointers they provide to other online sites will help you explore many alternative healing methods.

Alternative medicine

*Internet Resources on Alternative Medicine (gopher://
una.hh.lib.umich.edu/11/inetdirsstacks/
misc.health.alternative, Quantum Medicine (http://usa.net/qmed/),
Sumeria (http://lablinks.com/sumeria)*

For an excellent overview of nonconventional therapies, read Internet Resources on Alternative Medicine, a guide written by John S. Makulowich. You'll find a listing of alternative medicine resources grouped by type, namely, newsgroups, discussion groups, gopher servers, and Web pages. The list is extensive, covering more topics and sites than discussed in this chapter.

Sumeria provides an overview of alternative health and medicine. This Web site includes information on oxygen therapies (including ozone, hydrogen peroxide, hyperbaric oxygen therapy, and free radical treatment); herbal remedies; midwifery and other childbirth and parenting topics; aging reversal and rejuvenation; and alternative treatments and theories for AIDS, cancer, and immune disorders. Sumeria also discusses alternative science and technology, such as that provided by Mind Gear Inc. To keep track of changes on Sumeria, you can send e-mail to sumeria-announce-request@werple.mira.net.au with the word SUBSCRIBE as the message body.

The Quantum Medicine page covers electrophysiological reactivity, natural medicine, naturopathy, homeopathy, bioenergetics, acupuncture, and electroacupuncture. Quantum Medicine is sponsored by Hippocampus, Inc. (Hungary), the College of Practical Homeopathy (England), and the Association of Applied Quantum Bio-Technologies (New Mexico). You'll find discussions of clinical and scientific studies and links to related resources. The documents are comprehensive and well-referenced.

You'll also find many Usenet newsgroups featuring alternative medicine topics. For broad coverage of the field of alternative medicine, check out misc.health .alternative. You'll find detailed postings about aromatherapy, alternative treatment clinics around the world, explanations of chiropractic therapy, eye exercises, and nutritional supplements. You'll also find dedicated members who check into and report on the validity of various posted claims. Other newsgroups to consider include alt.folklore.science and alt.hypnosis. On Fidonet, tag Bodywork (healing touch, massage techniques, and recent developments in the field); Vheal (vibrational healing, therapeutic baths, aromatherapy, homeopathy, uropathy, radionics, dowsing, magnets, and crystals); and Norml (use of medicinal marijuana for a variety of conditions).

Ancient healing techniques

alt.health.ayurveda, OrMed WWW Page
(ftp://ftp.cts.com/pub/nkraft/ormed.html),
Spiritual Consciousness (http://www.protree.com/Spirit.html)

For information about spiritual healing, go to The Spiritual Consciousness page, also called Spirit-WWW. Here you'll find addresses for dozens of ancient heal-

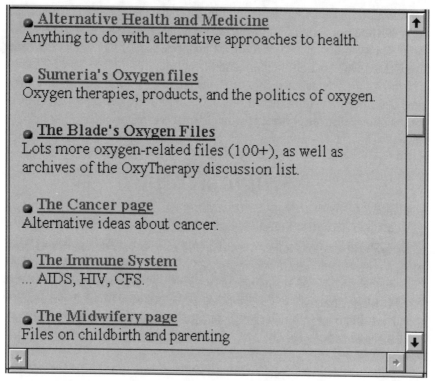

● **Alternative Health and Medicine**
Anything to do with alternative approaches to health.

● **Sumeria's Oxygen files**
Oxygen therapies, products, and the politics of oxygen.

● **The Blade's Oxygen Files**
Lots more oxygen-related files (100+), as well as
archives of the OxyTherapy discussion list.

● **The Cancer page**
Alternative ideas about cancer.

● **The Immune System**
... AIDS, HIV, CFS.

● **The Midwifery page**
Files on childbirth and parenting

Sumeria offers a good place to start your search for alternative therapies.

ing techniques that focus on healing the self or soul as a way to heal the body.
You can follow links to documents and resources dealing with channeling,
lightwork, reincarnation, auras, Ayurvedic medicine, chakras, hatha yoga,
pranayama, tai chi, Yan Xin Qigong, reiki, shiatsu massage, homeopathy, vibrational healing, foot reflexology, herbs, vegetarianism, and shamanism. In addition, you'll find the Kundalini FAQ, Pranayama Instruction, and Ayurveda
Resource Guide.

The alt.health.ayurveda newsgroup covers everything from ginseng to green
tea, with members posting questions and seeking advice for specific medical
conditions. Members discuss how to apply the underlying principles of
Ayurveda in a Western context. If you're looking for a trained Ayurvedic physician in your area, this is a good place to find a referral. On Fidonet, tag TCM
for discussion of theories and practices of traditional Asian medicine.

For a focus on Oriental medicine, try the OrMed WWW page and mailing list. OrMed discusses acupuncture, herbs, massage, breathwork, exercise, and more. The Web site includes mailing list archives, special files, the comprehensive OrMed FAQ, and other information about the mailing list. The FAQ gives an overview of Oriental medicine, explains the history of Chinese herbal medicine, describes what to expect during acupuncture treatments, and lists medical conditions that can be treated with Oriental medicine.

Aromatherapy

alt.folklore.aromatherapy, Aromatherapy-L (listserv@netcom.com),
Nature's Gifts (http://www.dircon.co.uk/home/philrees/fragrant/)

At Nature's Gifts in the United Kingdom, you can read about health and vegetarian diets and references to various books about aromatherapy. Nature's Gifts also provides a Guide to Aromatherapy, lists available oils, and explains how to use the oils in massage, baths, compresses, and steam baths. Similarly, the alt.folklore.aromatherapy newsgroup and the Aromatherapy mailing list both cover the use of oils for specific diseases and conditions and aromatherapy news.

Chiropractic

Chiropractic Page (http://www.mbnet.mb.ca/~jwiens/chiro.html),
Oregon Chiropractic BBS (503-224-4473)

John Wiens, D.C., has created the Chiropractic Page primarily as a pointer to online resources of interest to chiropractors, students, other healthcare practitioners, and the public. You'll find much useful consumer information on the Chiropractic Page, including press releases, descriptions of mailing lists, research summaries, MEDLINE search results, and information on how to contact chiropractic centers and organizations online and offline. The Web links cover everything from nutrition to body mechanics to headaches.

The Oregon Chiropractic BBS also offers chiropractic-related text and software files. In addition, you'll find conferences about legislative issues, workmen's compensation, health news and information, ethics and jurisprudence, nutrition, and herbal medicine, among others.

When I first started poking around the Internet late in 1991, the information I began looking for, naturally, was chiropractic-related. Unfortunately, my search was short-lived. There was very little information (in truth, none) on the Net related to chiropractic. That situation was unchanged until the middle of 1994. At that time, a couple of things happened. Chiropractors began showing up on the Net in greater numbers and interacting worldwide. In addition, my Internet provider began offering access to the World Wide Web through what is known as a SLIP connection. The first time I used the World Wide Web browser Mosaic I was absolutely hooked. The way Mosaic presented information graphically rather than as simple text opened up a new world of possibilities.

The World Wide Web is truly interactive. It allows an individual to act not only as a consumer of information, but as a provider as well. This facility gave me an opportunity to fill a void of chiropractic information that existed at that time by creating and maintaining the Chiropractic Page. The page exists to disseminate healthcare information, much of it provided by other chiropractors and healthcare professionals. The Web makes it incredibly simple for the consumer of healthcare information to find answers to general or specific questions he or she might have.

To give an example directly from the Chiropractic Page, one of the most common injuries sustained in the age of information is called repetitive strain injury (RSI), which can be caused by improper keyboard use. The Chiropractic Page offers a link to the Repetitive Strain Injury Page, which has information on the prevention and treatment of this common disorder. The Chiropractic Page also has links to a number of mailing lists and FAQ lists that offer support for a wide variety of healthcare complaints, such as headache, fibromyalgia, and chronic fatigue syndrome.

You can see that the future of healthcare is likely to look much different from today. The ability of the healthcare consumer to gather information about his or her own condition and apply that information to his or her own healthcare helps tilt the responsibility of individual healthcare back to the individual, where it belongs.

John Wiens, D.C.
Winnipeg, MB, Canada
http://www.mbnet.mb.ca/~jwiens/chiro.html

Complementary healthcare and natural medicine

*AlterNet BBS (508-827-5274),
Complementary Medicine Home Page (http://
galen.med.virginia.edu/~pjb3s/ComplementaryHomePage.html),
Natural Medicine, Complementary Health Care and
Alternative Therapies (http://www.amrta.org/~amrta), Paracelsus
(majordomo@teleport.com)*

The Complementary Medicine Home Page represents Dr. Peter Bower's efforts to catalog and facilitate research being carried out worldwide in complementary medicine. The site offers information on specific complementary practice topics, including acupuncture, reiki, shiatsu, reflexology, qigong, Ayurvedic medicine, homeopathy, chiropractic, and many others. You'll also find explanations of various alternative therapies, Branches (the Institute's newsletter), and links to related sites on the Internet.

If you're looking for a bulletin board with complementary healthcare information, try AlterNet. You'll access at least six conferences, including Health Consciousness, a bimonthly magazine with the latest in complementary medicine; Common Ground, a monthly newsletter with valuable health information; and The Family News, a quarterly gazette about oxygen information and products. Among the file directories you'll find a comprehensive list of FDA bulletins and other documents addressing a wide range of issues.

Although limited to healthcare professionals, Paracelsus, created by the Alchemical Medicine Research and Teaching Association (AMRTA), focuses on the clinical practice of natural medicine, alternative therapies, and complementary healthcare. AMRTA also offers Natural Medicine, Complementary Health Care and Alternative Therapies on the Web.

Herbal therapy

alt.folklore.herbs,
Herbal Hall (http://www.crl.com/~robbee/herbal.html),
Medicinal Herb Archives (gopher://sunsite.unc.edu/
11/.pub/academic/medicine/alternative-healthcare/)

You can join a lively discussion of herbs and medicinal plants on alt.folklore. herbs. Topics include the safety of herbs in pregnancy, use of herbs and medicinal plants for specific disorders, and several related issues, such as ethnobotany, phytochemicals, and herb gardening. You can also read the FAQ for Medicinal Plants by Henriette Kress and several other group members. It covers various herbs and plants, books and magazines about herbal medicine, and several online resources. At the Medicinal Herb Archives, you'll find text and graphic files about the Herb Research Foundation, herbs and herbal medicine, herbal medical contraindications, mail order information, and many other related topics.

- Medicinal Herb Garden
- Australian National Botanic Gardens
- Nootropic Page from Finland
- Longevity Herbs-Adaptogens-Nutritives
- Homeopathic Page
- FDA (login as BBS)
- Compressed <.zip> files
- Amrta Home Page
- Ibis Home Page Download a demo of the IBIS software
- AP news wireHerbNews
- WildCrafter's Barrow A Source of Adaptogenic and Nutritive Herbs

Learn why herbs are not just for seasoning.

Rob Bidleman's Herbal Hall provides the Herbal@crl resource files, links to several related sites, an opportunity to search the Associated Press wire service, and a huge page of links to an eclectic group of Web sites. You can read fact sheets about herbs and related products, including ginseng, schizandra, bilberries, astragalus, Ho Shou Wu, Reishi mushrooms, Fu Ling, and Gotu Kola.

Holistic medicine

Good Medicine (http://none.coolware.com/health/good_med),
Holistic (listserv@siucvmb.siu.edu)

Good Medicine is a bimonthly magazine that seeks to integrate holistic and traditional medicine to provide what it calls "preventive medicine for better health." The Internet version of the magazine includes samples from the complete printed version, offering several full-text articles with graphics. One issue explored aromatherapy, fitness, Hanna somatic education, massage, herbology, and psychotherapy. The Holistic discussion group provides a forum for holistic healing. Topics include meditation, diet, bodywork, yoga, acupuncture and acupressure, visualization, hypnosis, and biofeedback, among others. You'll find a similar group with the same name on Fidonet.

The Usenet news group sci.med is an interesting place on the Net for medical professionals to visit. It provides insights into the experiences and beliefs of laypersons both as they interact with the medical system and as they avoid it and move toward alternative therapies.

Patients posting on sci.med frequently ask questions that clearly should have been discussed in depth with their physicians. Medical professionals reading sci.med cannot help but get a sense of the hunger for knowledge that some patients have as they leave their doctors' offices. It's a constant reminder of how easy it is for doctors to fail to provide adequate information to patients. The knowledge gap between patients and medical professionals also results in frequent postings from people who are just looking for confirmation that what their doctors told them actually makes sense and conforms to a standard of care. It's a kind of electronic second opinion.

Practitioners of scientific medicine might have difficulty comprehending the attractions of alternative therapies. In reading sci.med, I have been confronted with both the tremendous scope of alternative beliefs and the wishful thinking that seems to underlie many of these beliefs. Many practitioners of alternative therapies post to sci.med, and it has been an enlightening experience to realize that most appear to be true believers in their therapies. At the same time, it has been apparent that a lack of basic grounding in principles of therapeutic evaluation and clinical trials has left these practitioners unable to evaluate which, if any, of their therapies are beneficial. I have found the discussions about alternative therapies in sci.med invaluable in discussing these same therapies with my patients when they tell me they are considering using them.

As with most Usenet groups, before starting to post it's a good idea to read the group for a while to get a sense of the personalities and topics under discussion. It's also important to remember the limitations of dealing with people via the Net. Flame wars can erupt unexpectedly, people might misrepresent themselves, and motivations might be obscure. Similar problems can occur to varying degrees in the real world. But in the virtual world of the Net without face-to-face interactions, these problems are heightened. A medical professional can have an enjoyable experience participating in sci.med, particularly if he or she maintains a sense of humor.

David Rind, M.D.

Homeopathy

Homeopathic Internet Resources List
(ftp://antenna.apc.org/pub/homeo/resource.lst), Homeopathic
Remedies FAQ (http://community.net/~neils/faqhom.html),
Homeopathy (homeopathy-request@dungeon.com), Homeopathy
Home Page (http://www.dungeon.com//~cam/homeo.html)

As the name implies, The Homeopathic Internet Resources List, created by Emiel van Galen, M.D., offers descriptions and addresses of the major homeopathic resources. The Resources List is updated regularly and provides online and offline addresses for homeopathic networks, libraries, private collections (of homeopathic references), and research centers. It also offers databases, medical journals, mailing lists, newsgroups, Web pages, software, pharmaceutical companies, and organizations.

For an explanation of homeopathic remedies, check the Homeopathic Remedies FAQ, maintained by Neil Sandow, Pharm.D. The FAQ features abstracts from the medical literature, provides the text version of the Internet List of Homeopathic Resources, and lists additional places for more information on homeopathy. Of particular interest is the full text of a Lancet article published in 1994, "Is Evidence for Homeopathy Reproducible?"

Another good homeopathy resource is the Homeopathy Home Page. You'll find a listing of homeopathy resources in the United States and the United Kingdom, a FAQ explaining the principles of homeopathy, organizations to help you find a homeopathic physician, suggested books to read, and information about two holistic mailing lists and the misc.health.alternative newsgroup. While you're here, you can join the Homeopathy list, an unmoderated discussion group covering all aspects of homeopathic medicine.

Meditation

alt.meditation, alt.meditation.transcendental, Meditation Archives
(ftp://sunsite.unc.edu/pub/academic/medicine/
alternative_healthcare/discussion-groups/newsgroups/alt.meditation)

The alt.meditation newsgroup compares meditation with medication for treating various medical disorders, debates New Age and metaphysical issues, reviews books on meditation, and discusses a variety of related topics, such as Eastern religions, tai chi, yoga, martial arts, and nootropics (cognition enhancers). The group maintains a directory of its archives at the sunsite.unc.edu FTP site. You can also join the Meditation echo on Fidonet or the alt.meditation.transcendental newsgroup. The TM Research FAQ (posted regularly as ten separate articles in alt.meditation.transcendental and forwarded to sci.med) contains research information on transcendental meditation and other health and educational programs founded by Maharishi Mahesh Yogi.

Neurotechnology

Mind Gear Inc. (http://www.netcreations.com/mindgear/),
Mind-L (listproc@gate.net)

At the Mind Gear Inc.'s commercial site, you can learn about mind machines and neurotechnologies, including biofeedback, light and sound brain-wave synchronization, and cranial electrical stimulation. The site also lists resources for psychoactive tapes, smart drugs, smart nutrients, and other related products. The Mind-L discussion group also addresses mind-altering techniques in general, and mind machines and biofeedback equipment in particular. Related topics include smart nutrients, hypnosis, relaxation techniques, and subliminal tapes and videos. You'll find serious research discussed alongside personal observations and freely shared opinions. If you want to look at archived issues first, check out the FTP site at asylum.sf.ca.us.

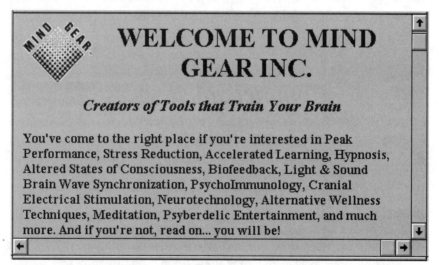

Be sure to use your head when looking for online information.

Vision improvement

International Society for the Enhancement of Eyesight
(http://silver.ucs.indiana.edu/~aeulenbe/)

The International Society for the Enhancement of Eyesight Web site describes vision improvement self-help books, research on myopia control, the role of bilberry in vision improvement, and the history of this field. You can also view an eye chart (RTF format), read the Natural Vision FAQ, and use links to go to the University of California, Berkeley School of Optometry and the Indiana University School of Optometry's EYEbase. The Natural Vision FAQ defines many vision problems and discusses dozens of components of vision therapy.

Women's health

Kristi's PMS Page (http://www.ccnet.com/~diatribe/pms.html)

At Kristi Weyland's PMS Page, you'll find herbal therapy, aromatherapy, and other alternative treatments for premenstrual cramps, breast tenderness, fatigue, acne, and related symptoms. You'll also learn about natural treatments for vaginal infections, bladder infections, and birth control. The site provides links to other Web pages and related newsgroups as well.

Commercial services
CompuServe

go BIORHYTHM Use personalized biorhythm charting to determine your emotional, mental, and physical states.

go HOLISTIC ($) The Holistic Health Forum (which prefers not to use the term *alternative medicine*) offers a place to discuss all aspects of holistic health. You'll find discussions in several message sections covering everything from Ayurvedic medicine to vitamin therapy. Political and consumer advocacy issues are also discussed. The forum permits commercial postings, so you'll see several retailers, manufacturers, and distributors online. The forum schedules both hosted and informal conferences. Often you can join a study group, like one for homeopathy.

Each section of the forum announces new library additions of software, text files, and graphics. Expert in holistic health, the forum sysops include physicians, scientists, chiropractors, computer scientists, and pharmacists.

go NEWAGE ($) CompuServe's New Age Forum offers information on yoga, natural healing foods and herbs, meditation, and mind-body interactions. However, the Holistic Health Forum will probably give you more specific health information than you'll find in the New Age Forum.

Delphi

go CUSTOM 153 The Homeopathic/Holistic Health Forum focuses on alternative healthcare options, including recommendations from members about where to find practitioners in your area. You can also access related newsgroups and gopher servers.

go GR NEW AGE The New Age Network, managed by Nama, features seven general categories: General Information, Astrology, Tarot, Humor, Oracles, Meditation, and Master Mind. Meditation covers techniques for meditating and its benefits, while Master Mind addresses the higher mind, visualization, and healing through the power of the mind. In the General Information database, you'll find information on many alternative health issues. Forum discussions cover the full range of New Age topics, from moon signs to chakras.

e•WORLD

shortcut TNC The Natural Connection (TNC) serves as e•World's natural health and holistic lifestyle center, with information about acupuncture, reflexology, Ayurvedic therapy, massage, personal development, and much more. Developed by Inspiration Associates, Inc., TNC features The Natural Kitchen (gourmet advice from chefs, healthful take-out restaurants, recipe swapping board); Holistic Resource Center (holistic health professionals and services, health foods resources, educational resources, a holistic fitness guide, reference library, file exchange); The Wellspring (for informal chatting); TNC Mini-Mall (catalog shopping, holistic classified advertisements, TNC Bookstore); an events calendar;

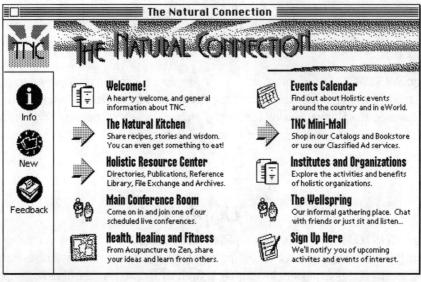

e•World's The Natural Connection brings together folks interested in holistic medicine.

holistic institutes and organizations; and a message board, conference room, and registration desk.

GEnie

keyword NEWAGE The New Age RoundTable is a lively place to find information and support for all alternative therapies. You'll find a category for Health and Well-Being topics. New Age professionals can discuss such issues as ethics, confidentiality, fees, nurturing oneself, and building a practice.

Prodigy

jump NEW AGE ($) Although the New Age Forum focuses mainly on astrology, psychic predictions, and other topics not related to alternative medicine, you'll find some discussions of ancient healing practices, biorhythms, and alternative therapies. However, you'll probably find more information on the Health Bulletin Board.

14
Disabilities

*P*eople with disabilities have benefited from rapid advances in computer and telecommunication technologies more than almost any other community. The use of these adaptive technologies has enabled individuals with disabilities to become more independent and less isolated from information and social contacts. In this chapter, we'll guide you to the best sites for information vital to people with any kind of disability. In addition, we'll provide both here and in other chapters key locations for information about many medical conditions that either result from or lead to disabilities. You'll also learn about rehabilitation services and strategies for overcoming challenges posed by disabilities. You'll find that disability-related resources are dynamic and constantly expanding, which is reflective of the rapid pace of technological development. For information and conferences specific to your area, be sure to check your local BBS or freenet.

Accessibility and adaptive technology

Clearinghouse on Computer Accommodation
(http://www.gsa.gov/coca/), Disability Resources
(http://disability.com/),
EASI (gopher://sjuvm.stjohns.edu/11/disabled/easi), InfoUCLA
(gopher://gopher.ucla.edu:4334/1), L-Hcap
(listserv@vm1.nodak.edu), National Library Service for the Blind and
Physically Handicapped (gopher://marvel.loc.gov/11/loc/nls),
Mobility (listserv@stjohns.edu), Trace Research and Development
Center (gopher://trace.waisman.wisc.edu/1),
University of Washington Disability Gopher
(gopher://hawking.u.washington.edu:70/11/disability-related)

Make the University of Washington Disability Gopher your first stop in any search for disability-related information. In addition to a wide selection of resources related to technology and disabilities, you'll have access to publications of Project DO-IT (disabilities, opportunities, internetworking, and technology) and the incredible DO-IT Guide to Disability Resources on the Internet. The DO-IT Guide features addresses and brief descriptions of mailing lists, electronic newsletters, newsgroups, Web home pages, and gopher servers. The DO-IT directory also stocks information and documents about chronic fatigue syndrome, deafness, blindness, adaptive technologies, the Americans with Disabilities Act, and offline resources for individuals with disabilities.

The Clearinghouse on Computer Accommodation, renamed the Center on Information Technology Accommodation (CITA), has a Web page that helps people with disabilities access electronic information about adaptive technologies. At the Clearinghouse Web site, you can learn about accessibility resources on the Internet, including mailing lists and gophers. You'll also find a listing of vendors who sell accessibility products and files about the Federal Information Technology Access Working Group and related agencies and programs.

Another important site is EASI (Equal Access to Software and Information), which has mounted many of its publications and other disability-related infor-

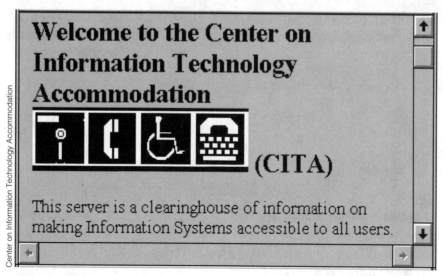

The Internet makes everything more accessible to people with disabilities.

mation on the St. John's University gopher. EASI should have a permanent Web site by now as well (try http://ultb.isc.rit.edu/~nrcgsh, the temporary site). As an educational resource, particularly higher education, EASI provides people with disabilities guidance in the area of information access technologies. At the EASI gopher server, you'll find a well-organized directory including Tips on Using Adaptive Hardware/Software, List of Adaptive Computer Products, and Recordings for the Blind. On the gopher server you can also read about EASI mailing lists and newsletters, publications by and about EASI, and the EASI journal, *Information Technology and Disabilities.* One discussion group (with a Usenet newsgroup gateway), the EASI mailing list, provides general information about adaptive computer access for people with disabilities, while the other discussion group focuses more on library access.

For anyone with difficulty reading printed information, InfoUCLA offers documents incorporating adaptive computer technologies, such as voice synthesizers, conversion into braille, and magnified on-screen text. The UCLA Library and the UCLA Disabilities and Computing Program are converting InfoUCLA documents into SGML (standard generalized markup language), which can then be converted into other formats used on the Internet. One such format is ICADD (International Committee on Accessible Document Design), which is used to help people with print impairment. The project's goal is to provide people with print impairment equal access to information. At this gopher server you can learn more about the project by viewing a demonstration of how InfoUCLA documents are converted into SGML and ICADD. You can also obtain InfoUCLA documents converted to ICADD.

The National Library Service for the Blind and Physically Handicapped (NLS), a branch of the Library of Congress, provides special services to the visually and physically impaired. The services include free loans of recorded and braille books and magazines, music scores in braille and large print, and specially designed playback equipment. At the FTP site (ftp.loc.gov/pub/nls), you can download the union catalog and other NLS publications. At the NLS gopher server, you can search and view these same documents. If you plan to use the system, read the documents at the gopher server that explain how the search and retrieval process works.

The Trace Research and Development Center investigates ways to make computers, other electronic equipment, and information systems more accessible to people with disabilities. To inform the public of available services, the Center operates a Web site.

Evan Kemp Associates maintains a Disabilities Resources Web page that offers a disability information tip of the month, a free consumer protection guide to wheelchair purchases, access to the Disability Marketing Group, the One Step Ahead newsletter, a comprehensive listing of other disability-related resources on the Internet, and a link to the Disability Mall.

Several mailing lists and discussion groups address the issue of access the mailing list. Mobility helps people with disabilities become more mobile by gaining access to opportunities in education and employment. You'll find the discussion engaging and the community wonderfully supportive as members share their feelings about disability, review new technologies, and meet other people with disabilities. The group also shares information about transportation and communication systems. L-Hcap and its Usenet gateway (bit.listserv.l-hcap) discuss medical, legal, and educational issues related to people with disabilities. Conversation often focuses on new and existing technologies, including adaptive computer hardware and software. You'll find articles taken from the Usenet newsgroup misc.handicap and from various Fidonet conferences. You can also tag Abled to join the disABLED Users Information Exchange, which provides information, help, and support for the disabled community.

Disabled helping each other get healthier on the Internet

If you are a person with a disability, you can find a lot of helpful information about your disability by joining one of the many Internet mailing lists focusing on specific physical or psychological disabilities. Autism, polio, cerebral palsy, amputation, multiple sclerosis, and depression are just a few of the numerous lists that thousands of disabled men, women, and children from all over the world are subscribing to electronically with their computers and modems.

A lot of online help is out there if you have a physical or mental disability. Whether it's a visual or hearing impairment, a neuromuscular disorder or paralysis, or even a spinal cord injury, there's an Internet special-interest list out there for you. On these lists, you can find the latest treatments for your disability or learn about the newest drug therapies. How do these drugs and treatments affect others with your disability? All these things and more can be learned and shared online with others, thanks to the Internet.

As someone with polio since age five, I use a respirator and a motorized wheelchair. I felt that many isolated, disabled people like me, especially those who were home-bound, could have a whole new world opened to them via telecommunications. In early 1992, I met with representatives from St. John's University, Grumman Aerospace, *Newsday*, and the Henry Viscardi School for the Disabled here on Long Island, New York, where I live. We talked about using computers and modems to network disabled people. I suggested telecommunications could open many new doors to those severely disabled men, women, and children who couldn't get to school or work.

Dr. Robert Zenhausern of St. John's University had already been sponsoring online special-interest lists for the disabled. Thanks to Dr. Z and St. John's, we started a new list called Mobility. Mobility was intended to be an electronic community center for disabled computer users. It would be an electronic meeting place and library where disabled folks from all over the world could find and share information and discuss all aspects of all disabilities.

By 1995, Mobility had about 300 subscribers from all over the world. Teachers in Hong Kong, disabled folks in Europe, and handicapped men and women from the United States and Canada were sharing and learning about everything from wheelchairs to healthcare. Then in September of 1994, Dr. Zenhausern let me start my Polio list. It has helped polio survivors in remote areas of the United States find doctors specializing in postpolio syndrome. Our Polio list subscribers have posted information on drugs that have helped others live more productively despite their polio. Everything from braces to cold intolerance to drug side effects has been discussed on my Polio list, which includes parents, family members, and doctors as subscribers. Together, thanks to the Internet, we are helping each other lead happier, healthier, more productive lives.

Robert Mauro

Amputees

*Amputee (listserv@sjuvm.stjohns.edu), Gimp Home Page
(http://www.primenet.com/~lathrop/gimp.html),
National Amputee Connection BBS (408-249-4852)*

The National Amputee Connection BBS, operated by Rob Thurlow, offers amputee support and also a forum for people to talk about living with amputated limbs. Among the conferences offered are Abled, Ablenews, Amputee, Abled_Athlete, Blinktalk, CFS, Chronic_Pain, CPalsy, Diabetes, Post_Polio, Rare_Condition, Silenttalk, Spinal_Injury, Survivor, Carcinoma, Ask_A_Nurse,

Grand Rounds, Bodywork, Holistic, TCM (Asian medicine), and VHeal (vibrational healing). If you'd rather keep in touch via e-mail, Ian Gregson moderates the Amputee listserv, which offers members the opportunity to exchange information, chat with each other, and share wisdom accumulated over the years.

On Douglas Lathrop's Gimp Page, you'll find a lot of useful information, including the full text of the ADA and links to Gallaudet University and the Cornucopia of Disability Information. Other interesting links include Canine Companion and the Archimedes Project, created to improve access to information for individuals with disabilities by influencing the early design of tomorrow's technology.

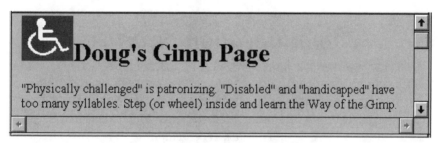

People like Doug Lathrop are opening new doors everywhere.

Blindness and vision impairment
bit.listserv.blindnws, Blindfam (listserv@sjuvm.stjohns.edu), Blind-L (listserv@uafsysb.uark.edu), Blindnws (wtm@bunker.shel.isc-br.com), Lowvis (listserv@sjuvm.stjohns.edu), Recordings for the Blind (gopher://r2d2.jvnc.net/11/Publishers_Online/)

Recordings for the Blind (RFB) is a nonprofit service organization that provides educational and professional books in accessible media to people with print disabilities. In addition to its audio cassette library, RFB offers on its gopher a listing of electronic books, which it calls its E-Text Collection. Here you'll find software documentation, reference books, law books, and works of literature. The e-text materials can be read with IBM-compatible, Apple, or Macintosh personal computers using the reading output method of your choice: braille, synthetic speech, or enlarged print. The gopher provides instructions for ordering items from the E-Text Collection, in addition to a list of contacts if you don't have the necessary hardware, software, or adaptive equipment.

Several discussion groups also offer support and networking opportunities. Blind-L focuses on computer use by and for the blind. Two groups maintained at St. John's include Blindfam, a forum to discuss the effects of blindness on family life, and Lowvis, providing support and information for people with visual impairments. The Blind News Digest (Blindnws) is an electronic newsletter that features questions, answers, news, and other information of interest to the blind community. Several Fidonet echos are also available, including Blindtlk, Blinktalk, and NFB_Talk (National Federation of the Blind news and discussion).

Communication disorders
alt.support.stuttering Mankato State University
Communication Disorders (gopher://gopher.mankato.msus.edu),
Net Connections for Communication Disorders and Sciences
(gopher://una.hh.lib.umich.edu/11/inetdirsstacks/),
Stut-Hlp (listserv@bgu.edu)

If you're looking for almost any online resource related to communication disorders, you're in luck. Judith Kuster's Net Connections for Communication Disorders and Sciences guide covers hundreds of online resources for communication disorders, speech science, speech pathology, audiology, and hearing impairments. The guide features sections about mailing lists, newsgroups, gopher sites, FTP, telnet, WAIS, and WWW. Within each resource type, she also breaks down the list further by topic.

Mankato State University's Communication Disorders gopher (in Communications Disorders directory under Academic Colleges and Departments) has established itself as the premiere site for information about stuttering. You'll see ongoing research projects, read messages from people who stutter, locate support organizations, and read about therapies for stuttering. You'll also find Thomas David Kehoe's FAQ for the Usenet newsgroup alt.support.stuttering. The FAQ contains background information about stuttering and provides practical advice for using the telephone and telephone company discounts for people who stutter. There's also a comprehensive guide for parents of children who stutter.

For additional support and advice about stuttering, check both the alt.support.stuttering newsgroup and the Stut-Hlp mailing list. In both discussion groups, you'll enjoy the ease and fluency of online conversation with hundreds of peers around the world.

Deafness and hearing impairment

Beyond-Hearing (majordomo@acbub.duke.edu), bit.listserv.deaf-l, Deaf Gopher Server at Michigan State University (http://web.cal.msu.edu/deaf/deafintro.html), Deaf Magazine (deaf-request@clark.net), Deafblnd (listserv@ukcc.uky.edu), Deafkids (listserv@sjuvm.stjohns.edu), Deaf-L (listserv@siucvmb.bitnet), Mrdeaf-L (majordomo@bga.com), Mrdeaf-L home page (http://www.realtime.net/~ref), Project HIIT: Internet for the Hearing Impaired (http://biomed.nus.sg/DF/databases.html)

You wouldn't expect to go to Singapore for information and support for the hearing impaired, but pack your cyberspace bags. At Project HIIT: Internet for the Hearing Impaired, you'll find the Internet Guide for Communication Disorders and Sciences, Deaf Magazine, Handicap Digest, Disability Newsletter, and ILRU Insights, which calls itself "the national newsletter for independent living." You'll also find links to several major FTP sites, including the Olivetti Archives for the Hearing Impaired, the Deaf Magazine archive, and the Oakland University Handicap archives. From the Project HIIT Web site, you can go to more than 15 gopher servers. You can also check to see what mailing lists and newsgroups are available, such as alt.sci.physics.acoustics, alt-support.stuttering, alt.support.tinnitus, bit.listserv.deaf-l, and comp.speech.

Even if you don't live in Michigan, Michigan State University's Deaf Gopher contains much information about ADA law, educational resources, electronic resources, bibliographies, offline organizations, deaf-related projects, Deaf-L and Slling-L (Sign Language and Linguistics) messages, and Deaf Alert, a collection of files about the influence of the deaf in history and culture. The gopher also has information about deaf-related technologies, camps, and learning activities. A separate directory lists organizations and services available to the deaf community in Michigan and nearby states. If you're looking for specific information for how the ADA affects the hearing impaired, look inside the ADA file for the Rights of Deaf and Hard of Hearing, provided by the Michigan Association For Deaf, Hearing and Speech Services.

Mrdeaf-L and the Mrdeaf-L home page, set up by Ron Morgan, specialize in information and services for deaf people who are mentally retarded. The discussion group includes teachers, parents, administrators, therapists, and allied health professionals. Most resources on the Web page are oriented toward education, but the site is growing and offers many links unique to this population.

The electronic Deaf Magazine keeps you informed about new online resources for the hearing impaired. You'll also learn about job opportunities, conferences, and other announcements of interest to the deaf community. The tone is friendly, positive, and practical. The large subscription base allows a lively exchange of information and opinions through letters to the editor.

You'll also find many discussion groups online. Deaf-L is for the deaf community and those associated with it. Deafblnd addresses deaf-blindness, while Deafkids offers a place for deaf children to interact. Beyond-Hearing features discussions of concern to both hard-of-hearing and speaking and lip-reading deaf people, especially members of SHHH and ALDA. On Fidonet, tag Silenttalk to join the Conference for the Deaf and Hard of Hearing, where you'll discuss hearing impairments, assistive devices, the Americans with Disabilities Act, and advocacy groups.

Developmental delays

alt.support.dev-delays,
Arc (http://fohnix.metronet.com/~thearc/welcome.html)

ARC is the United States' largest voluntary organization committed to the welfare of children and adults with mental retardation. On the Arc Web site, you'll find a series of fact sheets and publications on a variety of topics, or information about printed publications and how to order them. You can review the Arc Report Cards to the Nation on Inclusion, check Arc's Fetal Alcohol Syndrome Information Clearinghouse, read about people with mental retardation in the criminal justice system, and learn more about self-determination, family support, and aging. You can also jump to other disability sites on the Web or read (without links) an extensive list of disability-related Internet sites.

You'll want to join the active Usenet newsgroup alt.support.dev-delays to share experiences, read research updates and other information, and seek help coping with the challenges posed by developmental delays. You might also want to check the Our-Kids group reviewed in chapter 9, *Neurologic disorders*, under *Cerebral palsy*.

Discussion groups

Dadvocat (listserv@ukcc.uky.edu), Dis-Sprt (listserv@stjohns.edu),
E-clips (danyaon@savvy.com), misc.handicap,
Talkback (listserv@sjuvm.stjohns.edu)

Many disability discussion groups are available, including misc.handicap, which is extremely active and full of information, support, and good humor. You'll find several newsletters and digests posted here, along with messages informing members of new online resources. You'll also find discussion of adaptive technologies, educational and employment opportunities, and ways to bring down remaining barriers. On Fidonet, tag Ablenews for general-interest information (news, resources, referrals) for the disabled, their families, and professionals who work with them.

You might also want to subscribe to E-clips, a monthly compilation of news items, tidbits, and other materials gleaned from more han 640 print publications for the disabled (type *REGISTER E-CLIPS* in the subject line and *REGISTER E-CLIPS firstname lastname date* in the message body). Dozens of mailing lists (some covered elsewhere in this chapter) are available for discussion and information exchange. Talkback is one of several forums at St. John's devoted to children with disabilities. You'll also find Dis-Sprt, a discussion group for parents and people involved with parents of children with disabilities. Dadvocat offers an opportunity for fathers of children with disabilities or special health needs to share information, inquiries, ideas, and opinions.

What BBSing means to me

I had my first partial laminectomy in 1982 because of a ruptured L4/L5 disk. The second partial laminectomy was in 1988 after the same disk reruptured. Then in 1990 I had a spinal cord stimulator implanted for chronic pain in my lower back and down the back of my legs. Although the spinal-cord stimulator afforded me *some* relief, it wasn't as much as my neurosurgeon and I had hoped for. The chronic pain made me depressed. Disabled by two failed back surgeries, I had begun to feel pretty useless.

Then I discovered the wonderful world of BBSing! As we all do, I lurked on the BBS, just reading messages for a while. Then one message, from a man who wrote life wasn't worth living, hit home. He expressed his desire to end his life and told how he even bought a book on ways to commit suicide. I took it as a plea for help. Having had those feelings myself, I couldn't ignore him.

I wrote a long message back letting him know that he "was not alone." I told him how I had even written a suicide letter to my husband about how I couldn't take the pain anymore and how I felt he would be better off without me. I told the message writer how useless I once felt. Then I told him how I started laughing after I finished the letter because I thought: "I can't kill myself—I'll miss the last episode of Dallas!"

I waited on pins and needles for his reply. When I finally received his message, he told me how wonderful it was of me to share my thoughts and that he didn't think he could kill himself either. This was the beginning of my life changing for the better. I felt useful! I felt needed! I had found a place where people were just like me.

It didn't matter that some people were in wheelchairs and others weren't. We all had something in common. We could gripe all we wanted and know that everyone understood our moods. We exchanged our experiences with doctors and pain clinics. We all gave advice, shared support, and helped each other as much as we could.

I sometimes tell people that BBSing has literally saved my life. Had I not had the outlet of expressing my feelings and helping others, I don't know what kind of person I might be today. I have had the opportunity, through this electronic medium, to spread a little sunshine and hopefully make others laugh. I can share myself with others and, in turn, share in their lives. The BBS community is indeed a close-knit family, and a family of which I am proud to be a part.

I no longer feel alone. Quite the contrary, I feel needed. Imagine . . . I owe it all to something as simple as writing a message.

Linda Cummings
Mobile, Ala.

Rehabilitation

*Electronic Rehabilitation Resource Center
(gopher://sjuvm.stjohns.edu/11/disabled), National Rehabilitation
Information Center (gopher://val-dor.cc.buffalo.edu/11/.naric),
Occupational Therapy-Physical Therapy
(gopher://otpt-gopher.ups.edu/)*

If you're looking for rehabilitation resource guides, go to the National Rehabilitation Information Center gopher server sponsored by the National Institute on Disability and Rehabilitation Research (NIDRR). At the gopher server, you'll find descriptions of more than 400 NIDRR projects and research centers, details on how to request newsletters that document the findings of NIDDR-funded research, and, best of all, comprehensive resource guides for people with spinal cord injuries, strokes, or traumatic brain injuries.

```
NAtional Rehabilitation Information Center (NARIC)
Page 1 of 1

1    NIDRR Projects                                          Menu
2    Serials Survey                                          Text
3    NARIC Quarterly                                         Text
4    Rehab Briefs                                            Menu
5    Resource Guide for People with SCI and Their Families   Text
6    Resource Guide for Stroke Survivors and Their Families  Text
7    Resource Guide for People with TBI and their Families   Text
8    The Americans with Disabilities Act (ADA): A NARIC Resource  Menu
9    REHABDATA                                               Menu
10   Electronic Industries Foundation                        Menu
11   Who Tracks the Literature of Disability/Rehabilitation? Text
12   Publishers of Disability and Rehabilitation Books       Text

Enter Item Number, SAVE, ?, or BACK:
```

Not surprisingly, most disability-related resources are text-based for easy access.

The University of Puget Sound offers a central source of information on occupational and physical therapy. At the top of the gopher directory, you'll find a helpful document listing every resource available by menu title. If you're seeking rehabilitation resources, you'll find more than a dozen links. You can also read archives from several mailing lists, including ALS, EASI, GeriNet, Handicap Digest, Menopaus, MS, Parkinsn, Polio, Schizophrenia, Stroke, and TBI.

The Electronic Rehabilitation Resource Center at St. John's University offers a wide array of documents about rehabilitation. Directories include the following: A Glossary for Computer-Mediated Communication; Journals and Newsletters Database; National Clearing House for Rehabilitation Training Materials; Disability Awareness and Changing Attitudes; UN Human Rights for the Disabled; Assistive Technology for the Disabled Computer User; Bibliography on Assistive Technology; and a Dyslexia Database. Sometimes you'll find full-text documents online. Other times you'll find information about how to order printed publications.

Resource centers ·

*Cornucopia of Disability Information
(gopher://val-dor.cc.buffalo.edu), Disability Directory
(http://inform.umd.edu:86/Educational_Resources/Academic
Resources By Topic 79/Disability), Handicap News BBS (203-926-6168),
Handicap News BBS Archive (gopher//handicap.shel.isc-br.com),
St. John's University (gopher://sjuvm.stjohns.edu/11/disabled)*

If you want one-stop shopping for disability information, the Cornucopia of Disability Information (CODI) gopher server might be your best bet. CODI offers 22 main menus and several submenus to help you find exactly the type of information, support, and software you want. Resources include lists of disability organizations, directories, databases, hotlines, religious organizations, and sports organizations. You'll find statistics about disabilities; a collection of government documents covering legislation and regulations; a list of local, state, and national TDD phone numbers; a primer in plain language for people interested in learning more about disabilities; information about adaptive computer hardware, software, and other tools and appliances for daily use; directories of legal assistance; several membership lists for various organizations and committees; and announcements of conferences, meetings, and employment opportunities. You can use CODI to keep up with dozens of online resources (FTP sites, BBSs, Web pages, gopher servers) and search bibliographic databases. For practical tips, you can read articles from newsletters and journals, the ABLEDATA fact sheets and resource guides, the Directory of Independent Living Programs, and the National Rehabilitation Information Center publications.

St. John's University in Jamaica, NY ranks as one of the truly special places on the Internet. Under Disability and Rehabilitation Resources in St. John's main gopher menu, you'll find documents and/or links to just about every disability-related topic. The gopher also has files about specific conditions, such as repetitive strain injury, chronic fatigue syndrome, Parkinson's disease, and acquired brain injury. At the St. John's site you'll find archives for several discussion groups, including AltLearn, Autism, CFS-Fil, Madness, and TBI-Sprt; FTP files from the Handicap News FTP Archive Index; the Handicap News BBS Archive; the Handicap Software Archive (University of Oakland echo of Handicap News); and Able Inform BBS. St. John's is the best place to check for a support group related to disability. There's an excellent selection of educational and teaching resources as well.

The Disability Directory offers newsletters, articles, resource guides, current laws, upcoming conventions, classified ads, reviews and announcements of new products, and links to other online resources. You'll find the complete text of the ADA, additional legislative information on both the federal and state levels, the Handicap BBS list, screen readers, the IBM Disability Resource Center guides, back and current issues of the Braille Monitor, the Braille Forum, and archives and articles from scores of disability-related discussion groups and newsletters. The Handicap News BBS Archive offers a collection of information about and sources for the disabled. You'll also find a comprehensive, international list of BBSs that carry conferences and/or programs for the handicapped (look for HCAPBBS.LST or HCAPBBS.ZIP). A listing system for the BBSs explains whether they carry the Fidonet Abled or Abled_Eur conference, the Fidonet Blinktalk conference, the Fidonet Spinal Injury conference, the I-Link handicap conference, the Chronic Pain conference, or the Fidonet Silenttalk conference for the hearing impaired. The listing also indicates whether the conferences are TDD-compatible or have ASCII files.

I originally became involved in online medicine, not as a health professional, but as a patient. In 1988, I came down with chronic fatigue syndrome (CFS), which left me basically housebound and which I continue to be disabled from. The online community was and is my lifeline to sanity. CFS is a terribly isolating disease, and I saw my friends drop away one by one as I became unable to meet social obligations.

Computer networks offered a way to have social contact with others in a form compatible with my situation. My illness has left me with severe sleep disturbances and cognitive problems. If the only time I was wide awake was the middle of the night, I could log on to my Internet site and read and post messages. The Internet doesn't care what time it is. Because contact was written, I could save messages for a time when I felt up to reading them. I could also read them over and over again if "brain fog" was settling in. And if I was having a particularly bad flare-up, I could read and post from my bed with a laptop computer.

The Net offers tremendous resources to disabled people. I found several newsgroups that dealt with one or more aspects of my medical problems. I could talk to people in similar situations and get tips and share information. It was people on the Internet who taught me how to access MEDLINE. Soon I was reading the very latest abstracts about my illness. I learned about books and other resources, and I was able to get recommendations and information on various doctors in my area.

As I became more proficient in using the Internet, I found that my nursing skills and information could help other people. This is very important to me. I loved being a nurse, and I was happy that I could find a way to maintain contact with my profession. The sci.med.nursing newsgroup allows me to talk to other nurses and keep up with what's happening in my field. The sci.med newsgroup keeps me informed about the latest advances in medicine.

But most important to me is that I can answer some of the questions nonmedical folks ask about health problems. This allows me to feel that my training can still serve some useful purpose to others, and that even if I can no longer work in bedside care, the training is not wasted. I also learned enough to start a medically oriented computer bulletin board of my own.

Camilla Cracchiolo, R.N.
camilla@primenet.com
Shrine of the Cybernetic Madonna BBS, 213-766-1356

Commercial services
America Online

keyword disABILITIES Whether you're an individual with a disability, a caregiver for a disabled individual, or a health professional, you'll find the disABILITIES community of the Better Health & Medical Forum a supportive and informative place to visit. Employers and employees can learn about the rights of the disabled worker and how to make the work place accessible to everyone. The Assistive Technology area shows how computer technology can fundamentally change what it means to be disabled. Here members can share their experiences with various products and talk about adaptive technologies, such as personal computers, speech synthesizers, computer software, and adaptive keyboards. The reading room is well-stocked, and in the library you'll find software and documents explaining assistive technology. Peter Green, a member of Apple Computer's Worldwide Disability Solutions Group (started in 1985), coordinates the Assistive Technology area and welcomes suggestions for new additions from online members.

CompuServe

go DISABILITIES ($) The Disabilities Forum provides a meeting place for people with all types of disabilities, their loved ones, and those who work to make their lives more manageable. You'll find a full complement of helpful, understanding sysops, all of whom either have a disability or work with people who do. Led by administrator Dr. David Manning, forum leaders encourage tolerance among all members. If necessary, sysops will delete inappropriate remarks and messages and lock out disruptive individuals to maintain a supportive and open atmosphere. Libraries and message centers address developmental disabilities, emotional disturbances, deafness and hearing impairment, learning disabilities, vision impairments, mobility impairments, government activities, education and employment, family life and leisure time, and multiple sclerosis.

go HUD The Handicap Users' Database (HUD) provides articles (including online reprints from *Accent on Living*, *The Catalyst*, and the *Disability Rag*), software and hardware reviews, a reference library, disability news updates, and Veterans Administration rehabilitation research. Sysops organize lists of disability-related organizations according to focus (advocacy, job training, self-help, etc.) and nature of disability (mobility, hearing, sight, etc.). You'll also find a link to the IBM Special Needs Forum, an alphabetical index to HUD documents and menus, and a list of new additions, often helpful to frequent visitors.

go IBMSPECIAL The IBM Special Needs Forum offers special education solutions to teachers, parents, developers, and others. You'll be able to communicate through the message board and the conference rooms with an international community of people who are using IBM products to overcome disabilities. You can also search an extensive file collection in the library.

Delphi

go CUSTOM 015 In the Handicap Forum, people with various disabilities can meet to share stories, trade tips, and learn about the latest technological developments. You can join several related newsgroups (including, of course, misc.handicap) and access disability-related gopher servers. Host Ginny Kloth and her cohosts encourage friendly support and learning online.

go CUSTOM 065 You must apply to join The Yellow Submarine, which is not a Beatles fan club, but a group of people with various disabilities and their friends, who enjoy being "not disabled" online.

go GR WID The World Institute on Disability (WID) created WIDnet to provide telecommunication and information services to people with disabilities, disability advocates, and others interested in disability policy issues. You can join several targeted forums, go to the Coffee Shop for general discussion and debate, search the resource libraries and job bank, access the major disability-related Internet resources, and take advantage of many other high-level Delphi SIG services. WIDnet also allows you to examine several databases, including ERIC, CODI, the Federal Register, NIDRR Grants, and the ILRU Directory. By now, however, WIDnet might have left Delphi to reside at its long anticipated Internet address (wid.org).

e•World

shortcut DISABILITY The Disability Connection brings together people interested in topics related to children and adults with disabilities, including many leading disability vendors and organizations. In Hot Off the Press you can read documents from the Parents Let's Unite for Kids newsletter, the RSI Newsletter, Home Automation Newsletter, the Disability Rag, and many other publications. The Assistive Technology section includes information from Apple Computer's Worldwide Disability Solutions Group and the Macintosh Disability Resources library. In Face to Face, you can view information from assistive technology vendors; visit the Special Needs Project Bookstore; and learn about Telecommunications for the Deaf, Inc., the Breckenridge Outdoor Education Center, the National

Rehabilitation Information Center, and the CPB/WGBH National Center for Accessible Media. You can also read Exceptional Parent Magazine, the premier source of information for parenting a child with a disability. On e•World, you'll also have access to a collection of six resource libraries; a Family Support Bulletin Board; news and information; and an online subscription card. The Trace Center Cooperative Library includes ABLEDATA, a comprehensive listing of products for people with disabilities; REHABDATA, more than 40,000 bibliographic records with abstracts of materials in the NARIC library; and the Trace Information Center, with documents on issues of civil rights, accessibility, funding, product design, and more. The CONET Text Library offers five basic categories of information: funding, laws (other than ADA), access, ADA details (very comprehensive), and other information (including stroke, chronic fatigue syndrome resources, and state programs). The Let's Talk message board covers many individual diseases and disabilities, including Fragile X Syndrome and other genetic disorders, polio and postpolio syndrome, posttraumatic stress disorder, fibromyalgia, attention deficit disorder, and spinal cord and head injuries. There are also discussions about mobility, access, social and political concerns, and advocacy.

shortcut MADENTA Madenta Communications, which develops and manufactures assistive software and electronic products, provides documents and a FAQ about its products, which include Telepathic, ScreenDoors, Pre-Dict-ate, RevolvingDoors, Magic Cursor, and the PROXi Environmental Control System. The company also provides the Madenta newsletter, a software library, and a message board where you can meet other users of Madenta products and suggest future product development.

Shortcut STTS Straight to the Source is the e•World forum where software and hardware companies provide information and support for their products and services. You'll find the latest product information, demonstration software, FAQs, and a message board for asking questions and sharing experiences. Vendors that offer assistive computing hardware and software include Madenta Communications, Don Johnston, Inc., and Berkeley Systems.

In addition, Apple Computer's Worldwide Disability Solutions Group maintains a comprehensive free database of information about Macintosh assistive technology products that provide more than 100 solutions for individuals with disabilities. You can search the Macintosh Disability Resources database by keyword, product name, developer name, disability type, or a text description of what you're seeking. Your search will yield product description and developer contact information. You can download the database from e•World (shortcut DISABILITY) and America Online (keyword DISABILITY). You can also visit the Disability Solutions Group on the WWW at http://www.apple.com/disability/welcome.html.

GEnie

keyword ABLE The DisAbilities RoundTable covers a wide range of topics through its bulletin board, software libraries, and real-time conferences. From here you'll also have access to the GEnie Public Forum and LiveWire Magazine. Topics for discussion include legislative issues, personal rights, employment and education, sports and leisure, adaptive technologies, visual impairment issues, speech technology and screen access, hearing impairment issues and tinnitus, and learning disabilities. You'll also find information about diabetes and chronic fatigue syndrome, locate an e-mail pen pal, test your knowledge of disabilities trivia, and talk about any issue in the open forum. You can discuss sexuality and disabilities privately in a category open by invitation only. Also be sure to visit the Equal Access Cafe while you're at the RoundTable.

15
Searching for medical resources

With medical resources spread all over the globe, it's not always easy to find what you want, especially on the Internet. If you're looking for answers to questions about cancer, AIDS, or disabilities, your job's simpler since several sites are devoted exclusively to these conditions. However, for many other diseases and disorders, information is scattered around cyberspace with bits and pieces on various gopher servers, Web servers, and BBSs. But Yahoo! There are shortcuts—Internet catalogs and guides like Yahoo that will take you where you need to go with the simple click of a mouse or the push of a key. Besides these index services, you can also use search engines to locate resources based on a keyword you supply. You'll also find plenty of links from any of the major resources discussed previously in this book. For example, as described in chapter 5, *General health information*, HealthLinks serves both as an excellent source for health information and as a search engine for tracking medical topics across the Internet.

CARL Corporation's UnCover
telnet database.carl.org

Many databases available at CARL require a password and licensing fee, but you can search some of CARL's library catalogs and databases for free. To search for health and medical references, select UnCover, a periodical index and document delivery service. Anyone can search UnCover for free, but delivery of documents is cheaper if you establish an account. You can search by name, keyword (from title, subtitle, or abstract), and journal title. The service provides user-friendly help. You don't have to pay for citations, abstracts, or summaries of any reference you find. If you decide you want the full text, the service will advise you of the delivery cost in advance (includes copyright fee).

EINet

Health page (http://galaxy.einet.net/galaxy/Community/Health.html), Medicine page (http://galaxy.einet.net/galaxy/Medicine.html)

On your journey through cyberspace, you'll find EINet Galaxy a good guide to worldwide information and services. Galaxy organizes information by topic, which makes searching quick and easy. Once you've selected Health, for example, you'll see a page with various links organized by subtopics, articles, guides, product and service descriptions, collections, directories, and organizations. By choosing any of these listings, you'll transfer directly to the online site you've selected. At the bottom of the Galaxy page is a search engine to comb the WWW, hytelnet links, and gopherspace with a keyword. As with many searching tools, however, you'll find many listings that won't be helpful, such as medical school departments and other academic listings, many of which are primarily for internal use.

Electronic Newsstand and Bookstore

gopher://gopher.enews.com:2100/11/health/pubs/

The Electronic Newsstand stocks academic journals, medical books, health newsletters, and other publications about healthful living and alternative medicine. For each you'll find a description of the publication, a current table of contents (often with a synopsis of articles), archives of the tables of contents for past issues, sample articles, and subscription information. If you subscribe online, you'll sometimes receive a discount, although the actual publication will arrive via U.S. mail. The Electronic Newsstand's Health and Medical

Center also provides links to many major online medical resources, in addition to information about newsgroups, mailing lists, and FAQs. If you go to the main menu of the Electronic Newsstand, you can search all menus by keyword. Accessible from the Health and Medical Center, the Electronic Bookstore has a less impressive menu than the Newsstand, although the Bookstore does include the full line of Williams & Wilkins medical textbooks. For each title you can read general information about the book, a table of contents, and a selection of text.

Gopher Jewels

gopher://cwis.usc.edu/11/Other_Gophers_and_Information_Resources/Gophers_by_Subject/Gopher_Jewels

You'll see references to the Gopher Jewels directory throughout gopherspace, but don't be disappointed when you get to the medical section and find only three relevant directories (Disability Information, Medical Related, and Psychology). The Medical Related menu will take you to another level, with listings of Nursing, Veterinary, and Medical Related (misc). Inside Medical Related (misc), you'll find links to medical schools and medical school libraries, health associations, government agencies, research centers, online magazines, and databases. The other directories offer similar types of menus for each specialty. At each level you can search the Gopher Jewels menus by keyword, probably the fastest way to locate what you want.

When the *General Practitioner* newspaper asked me to write a lead psychiatry article on seasonal affective disorder (SAD), I almost turned the commission down. What did I know about it? I'm a psychiatrist, but the concept of SAD was not part of my daily work.

Curiosity overcame me, though, and I thought I would do some research before accepting the commission. Textbooks implied that SAD was a "footnote" subject—once fashionable, now discarded and all worn out. A MEDLINE search trawled up relatively few papers, often based on research with only a handful of patients and frequently contradictory.

I posted the results of my researches in the mental health library of MEDSIG (a CompuServe forum) and requested help. Did anyone have new research or experience of having or treating SAD? A few helpful suggestions came back. Then a posting in some Internet newsgroups unleashed an avalanche of personal accounts, descriptions of research, and treatment of the disorder.

Armed with this wealth of information and current opinion, I felt able to tackle the article. After the article was published, enough colleagues and general practitioners contacted me to suggest that SAD was anything but a footnote subject as far as real-world people were concerned. Many responding to the article wanted to know where they could get light boxes (the bright lights that seem to relieve SAD in winter). Again, I turned to the Internet and its newsgroups, posting requests for the names and addresses of manufacturers. I now know every light-box manufacturer under the sun, and, what is more important, so do my colleagues and general practitioners treating their patients.

Dr. Ben Green

HealthNet

http://debra.dgbt.doc.ca/~mike/healthnet/

The Healthnet WWW Demonstration Project represents a major step for Canada in integrating Internet medical resources with its national healthcare program. The Project aims to inform policy makers, healthcare professionals, and the general public about potential applications for healthcare networks. You'll find many links to health information and resources across the Internet, including Lee Hancock's Health Resource List, Medical Matrix, and the Harvard Index of Medical and Health Care Resources. There's also a HealthNet FAQ. The site is bilingual, with information in both English and French.

HospitalWeb

http://dem0nmac.mgh.harvard.edu:80/hospitalweb.html

HospitalWeb is a network of several dozen hospitals linking individual Web servers. Most information offered at these Web sites serves as a hospital yellow pages rather than patient education. Still, you might want to use HospitalWeb if you're trying to locate a particular physician or other healthcare professional, or if you want to find what services are offered by specific hospitals.

Index to Medical Information

http://merlin.gatech.edu/lcc/idt/Students/Ruby/Home.html

Georgia Institute of Technology's Index to Medical Information is a straightforward, alphabetical listing of major online resources for just about every medically related topic available on the Internet. You'll find links for specific diseases, such as AIDS, cancer, mood disorders, and repetitive strain injuries, and links for broader topics as well, such as artificial intelligence, biochemistry, and informatics. You can also jump to other indices, such as the Virtual Library, Lee Hancock's medical resource categories, and medical gopher lists.

Inter-Links

http://www.nova.edu/Inter-Links/medicine.html

If you have either a graphical or a text-based Web browser, you'll find Inter-Links an indispensable tool for locating health resources. Through Inter-Links, you can fetch a document, jump to a directory menu, or start an actual program. The concise first layer of menus will take you to many resources, including AIDS and Cancer Information, Consumer Health Information, Health-Related Discussion Groups, Practice Guidelines, Health Resource List, Medical Matrix, Medical Resource List (Library of Congress), Resources by Medical Specialty (Yale Biomedical Gopher), HealthNet (Canada), and the National Institutes of Health. Inter-Links also offers a comprehensive listing of psychological resources, described in chapter 10, *Mental health and psychology.*

From gatekeeper to guide

What's the latest diagnostic tool for Alzheimer's disease? Is surgery necessary for prostate cancer? Are my children at risk for leukemia because we live near power lines? Where can I get current information on chronic fatigue syndrome?

I get questions like this every day. I'm not a doctor, but I've been a medical librarian for more than 14 years. Searching for medical information can be time-consuming and frustrating, and I've made a career of helping both physicians and laypersons ferret out medical information.

In the past I acted more as an intermediary. Much of the published medical, clinical, and research literature was, and still is, accessible through a variety of online resources. Although the actual information would ultimately come from a printed source—a textbook or medical journal—finding that source often involved complex searches using sophisticated search languages on different online databases. At the time, this required considerable training and wasn't for the faint of heart. Most physicians and laypersons deferred to a librarian to perform these literature searches.

I've also found myself acting as a proactive gatekeeper for others by developing a dial-up bulletin board system (BBS) that, among other things, offered a digest of medical information in the form of newsletters and bibliographies gleaned from a variety of online resources, including the Internet. Though no longer active, this BBS ran for nearly 10 years and was relied on by many laypersons who had no other easy access to online information.

In recent years, however, technical developments have changed my role from gatekeeper to guide.

While many of the databases that merely point to information (the index databases) still exist, more original source material is becoming available via the Internet and the World Wide Web—the same sort of full-text information you might find in a book, scientific journal, or government publication. At the same time, access provided by such tools as the Internet gopher and various World Wide Web browsers have made finding this information easier for the nonlibrarian.

Here at the University of California, Irvine, students and faculty have access to a bewildering array of online resources. Most make some attempt to use these resources that are available both on our local systems as well as the Internet. As access increases and users become more sophisticated in their use of searching tools, I and other librarians find that more of our time is spent teaching others to develop the skills they need to become successful information seekers.

As the adage goes, "give someone a fish, and he will eat for a day. Teach him to fish, and he will eat for a lifetime." We're teaching our users to fish.

Steve Clancy, M.L.S.
slclancy@uci.edu

Lycos

http://lycos.cs.cmu.edu/lycos-form.html

Lycos is a catalog of the Internet. The Lycos Web explorer searches the WWW daily to expand its database. Its index is updated weekly. You can use the Lycos search engine to find information about medical resources in its database. The search engine sorts the list of possible matches in descending order of relevance, and you can read a description of each match along with an excerpt from the site. Although Lycos doesn't offer a medical section to start your search, as EINet and Yahoo do, you can review potential locations before transferring. Your search will yield a list of titles, URLs, authors, and additional relevant information not shown by some other search engines.

Medical Matrix

http://kuhttp.cc.ukans.edu/cwis/
units/medcntr/Lee/HOMEPAGE.HTML

If you use a Web browser (text or graphical), you'll want to make Medical Matrix one of your first stops. The Medical Matrix is also available as a text document called The Medical List. You can use Medical Matrix as an annotated, online yellow pages to find (and transfer to) just about every health-related topic covered on the Internet. Health professionals of all specialties can use this site to keep up with important online resources. Medical Matrix also provides an excellent overview of the Internet and its tools.

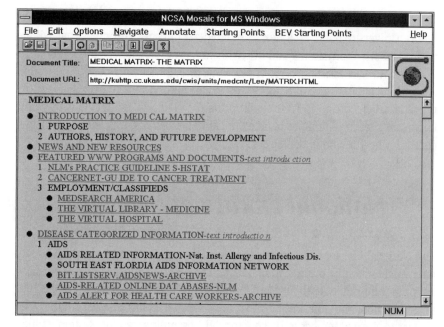

Two pioneers in online medicine, Lee Hancock and Gary Malet, maintain the Medical Matrix.

Medical Resource List

gopher://marvel.loc.gov/11/global/med/

The Library of Congress maintains a Medical Resource List that provides direct links to many online sites. While not exhaustive, the Medical Resource List does include most major medical resources, focusing on those of interest to healthcare professionals and researchers. You'll also find the latest guides to medical resources on the Internet.

MedWeb

http://www.cc.emory.edu/WHSCL/medweb.html

Emory University offers an index to Biomedical Internet Resources that will be most valuable to physicians and other healthcare professionals, including nurses and physician assistants. You'll also find directories with patient education links. Unfortunately, the directories don't offer descriptions to help you identify the most useful sites. MedWeb updates the list regularly and includes the most important sites for a number of fields, including bioethics, preventive medicine, consumer health, and toxicology.

National Library of Medicine

gopher://gopher.nlm.nih.gov/, http://www.nlm.nih.gov

The National Library of Medicine (NLM) is the world's largest research library for a single scientific or professional field. The NLM Web page and gopher server contain information about the Library and selected reference materials, but as is common, the contents of most journals and books are not online. The server does provide access to Locator, NLM's online catalog system, which searches for book titles and other resources on particular topics. For those with established accounts, the NLM server also provides access to MEDLARS (including MEDLINE), TOXNET, and three AIDS databases (no fee for searching). The NLM's Lister Hill National Center for Biomedical Communications offers Clinical Alerts and most recently the Visible Human Project, which maintains online an anatomically detailed, three-dimensional representation of the male human body (female to follow).

Using online dental resources

At a recent dental meeting, a local periodontist gave a presentation on a new product, a tetracycline-impregnated cord that's placed directly into the gum crevice for treating periodontal disease. As editor of our local *Academy of General Dentistry* newsletter, I wanted to include this topic in our next issue but didn't have enough material for a complete article. Two days later, I found a posting on dentistry@stat.com by Sam Ciancio, D.D.S., Ph.D., chairman of periodontics at the University of Buffalo, a world-renowned clinician and scientist. His posting included an overview of the product and how he has used it personally. He also answered concerns about safety. I had an up-to-date, rounded-out article that would have taken me several hours and several phone calls had I done it the old way (I wouldn't have had the time).

A patient with healthy teeth and gums complained of bad breath and a foul taste in her mouth for about an hour each morning after she awoke. After two nasal surgeries, the symptoms persisted, and she again visited my office to see if oral conditions were the source of her problem. Using Grateful Med I gave her a handful of references and pointed her to the public library. She found the answer herself. Tonsilloliths were her problem, a calcification on the tonsil much like gallstones in the gall bladder. Armed with journal articles, she had the diagnosis confirmed by her otolaryngologist. Now that she knows what's wrong, she's going to live with it for a while. At least she knows it isn't a hidden disease, such as cancer.

Another patient was distraught because of several unsuccessful attempts at quitting smoking. She became so depressed that she couldn't quit even in the face of poor health. Thanks to Grateful Med, I gave her several references for new ideas for treating depression that sometimes accompanies smoking withdrawal. With references in hand, she could then discuss the problem with her physician, who had been unsympathetic to her emotional needs. Her new perspective, a realization of the gargantuan efforts required for some people to stop smoking, allowed her to seek additional avenues of help. The last time I saw her, she hadn't smoked in two years.

Victor L. Commean, D.D.S.
President, Sinnissippi Valley Freenet Association
viccom@delphi.com, vicc@sinnfree.sinnfree.org

RuralNet

gopher://ruralnet.mu.wvnet.edu/, http://ruralnet.mu.wvnet.edu/

If you're concerned about the quality of healthcare in rural areas, you'll want to check RuralNet from the Marshall University School of Medicine. Rather than simply lumping all health science gophers into a multiscreen listing, the RuralNet gopher sorts healthcare resources into the following categories: Health Care Education, Health Science Libraries, Health Care Publications on the Internet, Clinical Resources, Patient Education Resources, Epidemiological Resources, Biological Sciences Resources, Computers in Medicine, and Health Care Policy, Reform & Management. The gopher server also has a menu of telemedicine resources, an emerging medium for delivery of rural healthcare services.

Thomas Jefferson University

gopher://tjgopher.tju.edu/11/medical

One of the best places to locate medical information is the Thomas Jefferson University medical gopher, which offers a well-organized directory. This server collects resources by type (mailing list, BBS, gopher, FTP sites, searchable databases, e-mail address, etc.); source of information (library, hospital, research center, government agency, etc.); and topic (cancer, AIDS, diabetes, obstetrics, dermatology, etc.). The server offers several powerful Internet searching tools so you can locate items of interest by either title or content.

University of Miami
gopher://gopher.med.miami.edu/

Like the Thomas Jefferson University gopher, the University of Miami server provides a well-organized menu to facilitate finding the resources you need. This gopher is the source of two enormous resource lists organized by discipline and disease that's offered in many other medical gopher menus. The General Health Sciences Sources directory features The Health Sciences Resource list by Lee Hancock and links to other library catalogs, medical software repositories, healthcare reform updates, health news-clipping databases, and several useful directories covering medical conferences, continuing education, job postings, and reference areas, among other topics.

Virtual Library
http://golgi.harvard.edu/biopages/medicine.html

If you want the ultimate shopping list for medical resources on the Internet, then go to the Virtual Library. Here you'll find resources listed alphabetically by name, with major subdirectories included as well. You might find other catalogs more accessible, but the Virtual Library is probably the most comprehensive. If you want an even larger database, then check another Virtual Library list called Biosciences.

WebCrawler
http://webcrawler.cs.washington.edu/WebCrawler/

WebCrawler, like Lycos, maintains an indexed database of material available on the WWW. The WebCrawler database is huge because it indexes the contents of documents, not just their titles or URLs. You can search this database with a keyword or words and receive a list with a numeric indication of relevancy (1,000 being the top score). WebCrawler is maintained at the same institution as Health Links (http://www.hslib.washington.edu/), and you can quickly transfer to WebCrawler from the Health Links site.

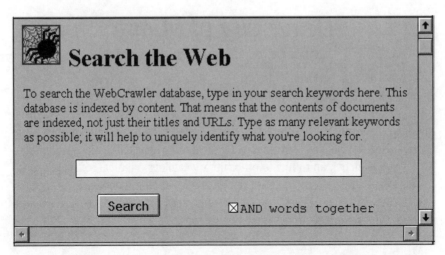

Search engines such as WebCrawler make looking for medical information easy.

Welch Medical Library

gopher://welchlink.welch.jhu.edu/, http://www.welch.jhu.edu/

At the Johns Hopkins University Welch Medical Library gopher server and Web site, you'll find links to many useful resources related to patient care, medical education, basic research, health news, and science writing. The Caring of Patients menus located here and elsewhere in gopherspace provide fine resources for patient care. Basic Science Research Resource is a collection of useful documents, searchable databases and catalogs, electronic newsletters, and discussion groups. The Welch server provides resources to help science and medical writers. Included are references to books on writing, improving one's writing style, preparing manuscripts for publication, and making effective presentations.

Whole Internet Catalog

http://nearnet.gnn.com/wic/med.toc.html

The Whole Internet Catalog, by Global Network Navigator from O'Reilly & Associates, provides links to a sampling of online medical resources. However, despite its name, the Whole Internet Catalog might not be as comprehensive as others, such as Yahoo, EINet, or the Virtual Library. If you use the Catalog to find a resource, you'll get a short paragraph describing the site and the Internet tool (gopher, WWW, FTP, telnet) needed to get there. If you're new to the Internet, the Whole Internet Catalog might be the most user-friendly place for your first online search. Categories include alternative medicine, cancer, disability, family medicine, healthcare policy, mental health, nutrition, professional medicine, safe sex, substance abuse, and U.S. and international health organizations.

Yahoo

http://www.yahoo.com/Health

You'll say exactly that when you find Yahoo, a hierarchical, subject-oriented catalog for the World Wide Web and Internet. Yahoo is probably the best place to start your Web search if you need online resources and information about any medical topic. Choosing the top layer of choices leads to many subtopics, some of which lead to other directories full of health-related resources. Yahoo provides descriptions for some resources, with direct links available for most. In addition to offering its own powerful Web-searching tools (with options for case-sensitive, Boolean, substring, and complete word restrictions), Yahoo can transfer you to other search engines, such as WebCrawler, Lycos, EINet Galaxy, Aliweb, and CUSI Search Engines.

Yale School of Medicine

gopher://info.med.yale.edu/1

As with many academic gopher servers, you can reach almost every medical resource on the Internet from the Yale Biomedical Gopher. Go to the Biomedical Disciplines & Specific Diseases directory and from there to the Other biomedical gophers subdirectory. Here you'll find more than a dozen options, including the opportunity to search comprehensive links to other online medical resources. The Yale server also features many news-clipping services found on other gophers, including citations and brief summaries of *New York Times* articles on medical subjects.

```
[ Yahoo | Up | Search | Mail | Add | Help ]                          ▲

Health: Women's Health

    ● Atlanta Reproductive Health Centre - information about
      infertility, endometriosis, contraception, menopause, and
      PMS
    ● Birth@ (8)
    ● Breast Cancer@ (3) [new]
    ● Crossroads Safehouse - a resource for battered women and
      their families. This site also contains information about what
      constitutes abuse and your legal rights if you have been
      abused.
    ● Endometriosis Mailing List
    ● Gynecological and Reproductive Health
    ● Kristi's PMS Page
    ● Maternal and Child Health Network
    ● Menopause Mailing List
    ● Obstetrics and Gynecology@ (2)
    ● Women's Health (HealthInfo gopher)
    ● Women's Health [dag.cc.columbia.edu]
    ● Women's Health Hot Line                                         ▼
 ◄                                                                 ►
```
Yahoo Corp.

Get ready to say Yahoo! when you arrive here.

Commercial services
CompuServe

go CCML ($$) CompuServe users can access the Comprehensive Core Medical Library, which contains current editions of major medical reference works, textbooks, and prominent general journals, such as the *New England Journal of Medicine.* You can search by subject, author, title, publication, or article type and retrieve a full citation, abstract, and sometimes full-text articles.

go HLTDB ($$) In Health Database Plus, which is updated weekly, you can retrieve articles from consumer and professional publications about healthcare, disease prevention, fitness, nutrition, health issues of children and the elderly, sub-stance abuse, smoking, and most other health-related topics. You can search Health and Fitness Journals for access to full-text articles from health publications, such as *American Health, Parents' Magazine, Nutrition Today, AIDS Weekly, Morbidity and Mortality Weekly Report, Patient Care,* and *RN.* You'll also have access to abstracts from several medical journals, such as the *Journal of the American Medical Association, The Lancet,* and *The New England Journal of Medicine.* In Health Reference Books and Pamphlets, you can search for informa-tion by keyword in publications such as *The Columbia University College of Physicians & Surgeons Complete Home Medical Guide.* You can also perform keyword searches in pamphlets issued by health organizations such as the American Cancer Society and the National Institutes of Health.

go INFOUSA ($) To learn how to receive free or inexpensive medical care and medications from federal and local offices, go to the Government Giveaways Forum. In the Health library and message sections, you'll read about obtaining free or low-cost health information and materials. If you're looking for information about clearinghouses, free books and videos, hotlines, and other offline medical resources, go to the Free Information From A–Z directory. You might be surprised at the quantity of materials available for even the most obscure medical topic.

go IQMEDICINE ($$) The IQuest Medical InfoCenter provides information about medical practice and research, pharmaceutical news, and allied health stud-ies through databases comprising journals, books, government publications, special reports, and many other published sources. You'll find IQuest's menu-based service easy to use, although you can bypass it to specify the database(s) you want to search. Depending on which database you select, you'll receive your results in the form of citations, abstracts, or full-text articles. Help (SOS) is easy to find and useful.

go KI ($$) Available to CompuServe subscribers in the evening and on week-ends, Knowledge Index is a service that offers access at reduced rates to more than 100 popular full-text and bibliographic databases. When researching health-related topics, you'll find the most useful sources of information to be three drug databases, nine medical databases, and two psychology databases. While some databases provide only bibliographic citations or abstracts, others provide full-text articles. You'll find the service flexible, allowing you to decide how much and what types of information to retrieve from various sources.

go NTIS ($$) The National Technical Information Service database references articles (usually with abstracts) from government-sponsored research, development, and engineering. You can search the database by subject words, author names, or the publication year. Health consumers won't find much useful information other than some health-related research projects or medical studies.

go PAPERCHASE ($$) PaperChase is an online information service that helps you search the National Cancer Institute's CANCERLIT database, the National Library of Medicine's MEDLINE, Health Planning and Administration (HEALTH), and AIDSLINE databases. By using PaperChase, you search all four databases at the same time, automatically eliminating duplicate references. While PaperChase is convenient and simple to use, you can search these same databases as easily by establishing an account with the NLM directly and using Grateful Med (see details later in the chapter). In addition, the NLM offers free access to three AIDS databases.

GEnie

keyword DIALOG ($$) GEnie offers access to the Dialog Database Center, which, through its more than 400 databases, helps you search for health, medical, and pharmaceutical information. Depending upon your search, you'll find articles from AIDSLINE, Consumer Drug Information, the New England Journal of Medicine, Consumer Reports, Drug Information, and Health Devices Alerts, among others. You can decide which citations to examine in greater detail and whether to view the full-text article (if it's available in electronic format). Before you search all DIALOG databases, you can practice searching a subset of the available resources at a reduced cost.

keyword MEDICINE ($$) GEnie's Consumer Medicine allows you to search the MEDLINE database, which covers virtually every biomedical topic. Consumer Medicine focuses on academic medical literature and doesn't index popular magazines as might be implied by the Consumer Medicine title. While you can practice using Consumer Medicine at a reduced charge (and with reduced access), you can also search MEDLINE and several other NLM databases directly by setting up a MEDLARS account and installing the user-friendly software Grateful Med (see details in the next section).

keyword MEDPRO ($$) If you want to search more than MEDLINE, you can use GEnie's Medical Professional's Center. Your searches here will access 15 major medical databases, some of which offer full-text articles. Included are AGELINE, CANCERLIT, MEDLINE, PsycINFO, the American Medical Association's Journals Online, Consumer Drug Information, the New England Journal of Medicine Online, and Smoking & Health. You can also limit the extent of your search to keep costs down. As with GEnie's other searching services, you can go to the Practice Area to try a less expensive dry run with a subset of available databases.

Grateful Med
MEDL ARS: 800-638-8480 (voice),
NTIS: 800-423-9255 (voice)

If you want to be absolutely sure you're keeping up with the latest medical findings in a particular area, you'll want to use Grateful Med software to access MEDLINE (MEDLARS online) and other online databases available through MEDLARS (medical literature analysis and retrieval system). Available for both DOS and Macintosh operating systems, Grateful Med performs simple and efficient literature searches that include the published abstract in 75% of cases as well as the full citation and keywords. You set up your search before signing on and read all retrieved information after signing off. That ability to work offline keeps online costs to a minimum. You can use another component of the software, Loansome Doc, to order full-text articles from a regional medical library.

– 283 –

To access any of the National Library of Medicine databases, you must first apply for an account with MEDLARS (call 800-638-8480). Setting up the account is free, and there's no monthly charge. Once you register, you'll receive a user ID code and password. You type these codes into Grateful Med once and never need to worry about them again. Because part of the objective behind MEDLARS and Grateful Med is to give rural healthcare providers access to the same information that a large university-based hospital would have, you're also given a toll-free number for logging onto MEDLARS databases. Although not essential for accessing MEDLINE, Grateful Med software is highly recommended. Grateful Med costs $29.95, which includes shipping plus *every* upgrade and new manual released thereafter, no matter how major the software overhaul. The program is available from the National Technical Information Service, at 800-423-9255. Specify whether you want the IBM or Macintosh version and have your credit

```
┌─────────────────────────────────────────────────────────────┐
│▓▓▓▓▓▓▓▓▓▓▓▓▓▓▓▓▓▓▓▓▓ HDL/Lifestyle ▓▓▓▓▓▓▓▓▓▓▓▓▓▓▓▓▓▓▓▓│
│      Enter your │  MEDLINE      ▼│  database search.        │
│                                                               │
│   AUTHOR/NAME │                                            │  │
│                                                               │
│   TITLE WORDS │                                            │  │
│                                                               │
│ SUBJECT WORDS │Lipoproteins, HDL Cholesterol               │  │
│                                                               │
│   2ND SUBJECT │Diet, Fat-Restricted                        │  │
│                                                               │
│   3RD SUBJECT │Exercise                                    │  │
│                                                               │
│   4TH SUBJECT │ │                                          │  │
│                                                               │
│ JOURNAL ABBREV│                                            │  │
│                                                               │
│   Limit to:  ⊠ English Language     ☐ Review Articles       │
│                                                               │
│   Include:   ⊠ Abstracts   ☐ MEDLINE References  ⊠ MeSH     │
│  ┌──────────────┐ ┌───────────────┐ ┌──────────────┐ ┌────────────────┐ │
│  │ Run Search ⌘R│ │ Find MeSH Term│ │Reference Nos...│ │Older Material...│ │
│  └──────────────┘ └───────────────┘ └──────────────┘ └────────────────┘ │
└─────────────────────────────────────────────────────────────┘
```

National Library of Medicine's Grateful Med
Software for the Mac (version 2)

Grateful Med will actually make you grateful for the federal government.

card handy. You'll receive an excellent manual with the software, along with technical support available by phone (800 number), by e-mail, or by an 800-access BBS. Online costs vary, but the average search costs about $1.25 (a complex algorithm is used to calculate actual charges). The average per-hour rate is approximately $18.

16
Rules of the road

*I*n part 3 of this book, *How to use online medical information*, we offer strategies for getting the most from your healthcare information quest. As you probably realize by now, you can tap into a huge number of online medical databases, libraries, documents, images, and resource lists, in addition to a lot of advice and support. You might find the resource possibilities overwhelming. To prevent overload, take the time to learn your way around, become familiar with different resources, and form your own personal strategy for searching medical information. Whatever your reason for going online, it's helpful to do some research in advance before logging on. While online, be thoughtful, considerate, and discriminating with the information you find.

Also remember that the Internet and other online services aren't one-way streets. If you expect to get help online, be prepared to give support and information in return. The bottom line is that people represent the most important online resource. How you relate in cyberspace will affect the quality of your experience and the amount of useful medical information you obtain.

This chapter starts you off by providing a basic set of rules. Cruising the information superhighway is no different than traveling on more conventional roads. Courtesy counts, and common sense is crucial. General Internet books address a much broader range of online rules, known as *netiquette*. We'll give you only the basics so you can get started.

Learn the ropes

If you've never been online, you might want to take a moment to consider what you'll find when you get there and how to interact with millions of other cyber-space citizens. Here are some tips for making the most of your online time.

Know your audience To learn the focus of any newsgroup, mailing list, echo, bulletin board, or discussion group you join, read messages for a week before posting any of your own. For example, the sci.telemedicine newsgroup gets many inappropriate clinical questions posted by people who don't realize the group deals with the role of computers in medicine. To avoid miscommunication, ask yourself these questions: Is the group composed of academics, clinicians, consumers, or a mixture of all three? What's the level of information the group provides? Is the forum educational, supportive, or debate oriented? Is the overall tone of discussion warm, professional, or humorous?

Read the group's FAQ or any other archives before posting a question The FAQ provides answers to common questions so group members can focus on providing support and more specialized information. You'll find the group's FAQ or a message about where to find it posted every two to four weeks. Some groups also archive their postings (or create a "best of" archive) and provide this address as well.

Keep the subject line for newsgroup postings short and to the point Imagine you're writing a headline for the morning newspaper and you want to catch as many readers as possible with the essence of your story. Also imagine you're doing a keyword search—what are the most unique and descriptive words related to your subject? Instead of writing "Having Trouble Getting to Sleep after Eating Porterhouse Steak," try "Insomnia after Steak Dinner." If your subject line is too vague or gets cut off, other people are less likely to read it. Depending on the group, you might want to add a parenthetical note to your subject line if your message is long, sensitive, or graphic in nature.

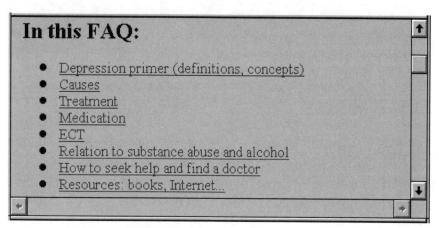

In this FAQ:

- Depression primer (definitions, concepts)
- Causes
- Treatment
- Medication
- ECT
- Relation to substance abuse and alcohol
- How to seek help and find a doctor
- Resources: books, Internet...

Be sure to check the FAQs before you ask.

Remember that the Internet is global Judgmental opinions about different cultures, countries, or people will provoke misunderstandings or downright hostility. Since English is the de facto language of the Internet, be understanding about the level of fluency of individuals trying to communicate in a second language. Think about how you'd sound asking a simple question in Japanese or Tagalog.

Use common sense when deciding what to include in your postings Don't post credit card numbers, passwords, social security numbers, or other confidential information. Unless you post anonymously through a special server, the message header will list your e-mail address, which you should also feel free to include in your signature. Group members will treat your postings with more respect if you identify any credentials you have (e.g., a healthcare degree or specialized training).

Help readers understand the context of your comments At some point, you'll respond to messages posted by others. To help group members follow your train of thought, include appropriate quotations from the original posting. If you respond to a few different sections of the original posting, type one quoted passage and then write your comments after each passage. Don't repeat the entire message, especially if it's long.

Use plain type Any formatting that you add will be lost when you send your message. You can show *italics* by bracketing the emphasized word in asterisks. Try to reserve all capital letters for very occasional shouts (HURRAY!). Typing in all capital letters is usually considered rude. One exception is on the disability-related discussion groups, where users access the network with a wide range of abilities, hardware, and software.

Reply to newsgroup messages via e-mail unless you're providing information or listing online resource sites of interest to others Some newsgroups and mailing lists exist mainly to share personal stories, in which case a posted anecdote is fine. However, when you respond to questions of a personal nature, it's best to answer via e-mail.

Finally, remember that thousands of people can read whatever message you post. Once you send a message to a newsgroup, you can't retrieve it.

Glance at this before you sign on

Understand your role You are neither a leader nor a follower on the Net. You are an explorer—a seeker and consumer of information. You are the ultimate judge of how and where to use the information. You should discuss what you have learned with your physician or practitioner. You might want to read other materials on the Net or off, or post similar questions in different newsgroups. You should combine Net information with your own experience, research, and good common sense.

Have reasonable expectations If you leave aside personal war stories (there are as many yawn-inducing bores on the Net as off), expect to get a relatively knowledgeable answer to a specific question. Don't expect a half-hour consultation. You're not going to find all your answers online. The physicians and others you meet don't have your medical history, your test results, or even your vital statistics. All they have is what you tell them. And they won't read through thousands of words to learn the subtle nuances of your condition or your new theory. So frame a specific question with only essential facts.

Understand the medical and scientific process There might not be a simple answer to your question, nor a consensus about which answer is right. Don't be concerned if one apparently credentialed respondent disputes the answers given by others. Challenge is a natural and common part of scientific learning. Read each intelligent response for what it is— an attempt to make order out of ambiguous or incomplete data.

It's just people on the other end of the line The physicians and others you talk to over the Internet are online for the same reasons you are—curiosity, an interest in talking to others, fun, and, in most cases, a willingness to help someone who seems in need. They're probably paying for their own time online, so don't make an impossible demand.

Be a framer, not a flamer The medical community rarely hides a miracle cure. Attacking others for their financial motivation in providing services won't get you information. In today's world, people work for money. Flames drive people off the Net when it's in everyone's interest to keep more people on. Even if you think someone's dead-wrong, try to frame a response with facts, not friction. Whether or not you convince the original poster, there are a lot of people lurking, watching your every word. You'll convince a lot more of them that you're right if you show them what's right instead of telling them your opinion.

Enjoy the special bonus The scientific and medical discussion groups often have unintentional humor. For example (from a discussion of safety glasses): "These glasses are capable of stopping a .22 caliber bullet at 100 yards (don't wear them when you test this)."

BZall@aol.com

What did you mean by that?

In online discussions, there's no body language or verbal nuances. You can't depend on subtle signals normally present during in-person or telephone conversations. Since you see only text, it's easy to miss a joke or misinterpret sarcasm.

You can reduce confusion by inserting a few typed symbols known as *emoticons*, including indicators for smiling and irony :-), winking ;-), and frowning :-(. Many general books about the Internet include a listing of these shortcuts, in addition to acronyms to cut down on verbiage. These include BTW (by the way), IMHO (in my humble opinion), ROTFL (rolling on the floor laughing), and FYI (for your information).

When researching medical topics, you'll also see many medical acronyms, ranging from familiar ones like BP (blood pressure) to terms that apply to a specific patient population, such as ESRD (end-stage renal disease) or ARDS (adult respiratory distress syndrome). Some acronyms are confusing unless the context is clear. For example, ADA can refer to the Americans with Disabilities Act, American Dietetic Association, or American Dental Association. If you see an acronym you don't understand, ask the person posting the message via e-mail for an explanation.

Not being able to see people online when you converse can lead to misunderstandings or flaming when one individual launches an aggressive attack on another individual. When responding in a critical manner to a posted message, you can defuse a flame war by saying "no flame intended" and including credible sources along with your response. Of course, it takes two to carry on a flame war.

Look who's talking

Would you take advice from a stranger on a bus? Or someone in a clinic waiting room? In the waiting room, for example, you might swap stories or share experiences. But even if that person had similar medical problems, you wouldn't necessarily follow his or her advice. Instead, you'd probably ask your doctor first to hear an informed opinion.

If after seeing your doctor you wanted more information, you could get a second medical opinion or go to the medical library to research the problem yourself. You might also want to speak to other informed patients with a similar medical problem, finding out what information they had, what experts they had seen, and what treatments had worked for them. Certainly before deciding on a course of treatment, you would want to get as much information as you could.

Participating in a newsgroup or mailing list, particularly unmoderated forums, is no different. If you follow the first piece of advice you get, it's like listening to that person in the waiting room or at the bus stop. What's different online is that you have dozens, maybe hundreds of people listening to your story. Some are real experts in their fields. Others have little expertise. Still others have biases that cloud their thinking or warp their analysis. Once you've joined a newsgroup, you need to follow the group for a while and identify the individuals who sound most reasonable and informed. Feel free to contact these seemingly informed group members via e-mail and ask them about their background and training. Most will be happy to talk. If you engage someone whom you respect, ask for references or other sources of information where you can learn more. Many health professionals will run MEDLINE searches to see if the peer-reviewed scientific literature is in accord with online claims. If you have Grateful Med or access to a MEDLINE account through a university or hospital, take the online suggestions as a starting point for your own research.

If you're really fortunate, some online contacts will offer to mail you articles that shed light on your problem. If the person you're querying isn't a medical professional but a patient like you, ask the same questions you would ask the professional. What are your sources of information? What references can you give me? What sites on the Net helped you? Above all, use common sense.

While you'll probably get most replies via e-mail, don't forget to check the original forum where you posted your message. One expert might post a response with which another expert disagrees. You never know when a simple, straightforward medical question will touch off a lively and informative debate. You'll quickly realize that good physicians with varying backgrounds and training can arrive at different conclusions on the same medical issue.

One other netiquette reminder. Always send thank-you notes. Even if you don't find a message particularly useful, thank the person who sent it. Keep in mind the mental image of a live conversation. Try to picture asking for suggestions at a party and then ignoring the person who responded to your request. You wouldn't do it in person. Don't do it online.

Evaluating medical information on the Internet: separating the wheat from the chaff

Patients have an almost unlimited source of medical information on the Internet and online services. Unfortunately, they also may have an equally large supply of misinformation. Several features of online communication promote the spreading of misinformation:

Anonymity Some people communicate under call names, some use pseudonyms, and some use their full names but misrepresent who they are (claiming to be a doctor or a patient with a similar problem).

Unbalanced contributions The postings that you read are put there by people who choose to participate in that particular newsgroup or forum. If people who favor one approach or treatment predominate, you might get a highly slanted perspective when it seems that "everyone is doing it."

Lack of accountability If you see a doctor, follow his or her advice, and come to serious harm, you have recourse both through the courts and through medical licensing boards. If following advice from the Internet harms you, your options are much more limited. It could be impossible to locate the person who gave the advice and hold him or her accountable. Furthermore, at the time of this writing, malpractice laws have not been clarified with respect to electronic communication. At worst, you'd have no legal protection. At best, you might be the first test case. Because of these potential problems, I suggest you assess the quality of the information you find on the Internet about a particular medical problem.

Several other tips:

Don't be afraid to ask the authors of postings who they are or what their qualifications or experiences are. The answers might not be truthful, but at least you asked. In a forum or newsgroup you might want to send the request as a private e-mail message directly to the sender, who might then feel less threatened and less inhibited about telling the truth.

Lurk in a forum or newsgroup for a while and see how other patients' postings are answered. Do the same people always jump in with the same advice regardless of differences in the questions asked? Are patients always directed to join a particular group or subscribe to a particular newsletter? Is the advice that the patient got from his doctor always wrong in the eyes of the forum members? If so, be suspicious that the group has been hijacked by a special-interest group whose interests might not be the same as yours.

Use the new information you obtain on the Internet as a starting point, not a finishing point. Gather information from various sources. Decide for yourself what makes sense and what you're comfortable with. Then discuss it with your doctor.

Daniel Shoskes, M.D.
Assistant Professor of Urology, UCLA

17
Getting results

Your online search for medical information won't always produce immediate results. Sometimes it will take a considerable amount of time and effort. The best way to shorten your search time is to develop an effective strategy. Whatever happens, don't get discouraged. You'll find someone, somewhere, who can help.

No one's paying attention to me

If you're not finding answers, maybe you're not asking the right questions. Whether you get results depends on both what you ask and how much preparation you devote to your research. People who take time to consider exactly what they need to know can write focused messages, usually no more than a few sentences long. These people will almost always get helpful responses.

To get results, it helps to list your question(s) as short bullets or numbered paragraphs that are easy to read. Usually the more open-ended the question, the less helpful the responses are. When looking for information, consider the following points:

➤ People online generally respond to requests for addresses of online (and offline) resources covering a particular medical topic. People are open to steering you in the right direction.

➤ You might not receive a response to a request for general information on a medical topic. If you ask a question like "What is lupus?" you'll be fortunate if you receive more than just a short description of the disease, perhaps from a knowledgeable patient who's done his or her own research. Usually vague questions produce vague, if any, answers. As previously mentioned, always look for a FAQ. If you have a common question, chances are the answer is in the FAQ of the appropriate newsgroup.

➤ Requests for well-defined information usually elicit one or more responses. A question like "What are the indications for colonoscopy?" is easier to answer than a personal question like, "Will my heart condition present any problems during the procedure?" Only a physician who has actually examined you and knows your history can answer the latter question.

➤ Requests for second opinions produce mixed results. The less information you provide, the less help you're likely to get. On the other hand, posting your life history will deter potential respondents. Rather than seeking a second opinion, lower your expectations. Use your medical contacts in cyberspace for information about specific issues that pertain to your problem. Don't look for an online diagnosis or a recommendation to proceed with surgery. Specific diagnostic and treatment decisions are more appropriate for a physician whom you see in person.

If you want information about a particular medical problem, make your request short and reasonable. Give a one-paragraph summary of your current condition and simple test results, such as blood chemistry, urinalysis, or other relevant information. Acknowledge in your message that you realize the limitations of online medical advice (that will relieve potential respondents of worries that you expect a cyberspace diagnosis or prescription for treatment). Offer to send more information about your medical history via e-mail to anyone generous enough to respond. Remember: If you post the initial message in a newsgroup, hundreds of people might read your personal medical history.

Requests for emergency assistance have no place online. In active forums, particularly those on commercial services, you might get a rapid response, but you won't have time to consider whether the suggestion is credible. An offline hotline (such as a poison control center) is better equipped to respond quickly and appropriately. Best of all, call your personal physician. Healthcare professionals who recognize a true emergency online might send a "get thee to an emergency room" reply, but don't count on this and never use the Internet or any commercial online service as an emergency room. Also, keep in mind that the newsgroups and Web sites identified as emergency medical locations are actually forums for emergency medical personnel to discuss professional issues. These forums are not alternatives to calling 911.

One possible exception is the case of suicidal thoughts. People who post desperate messages and pleas for help and support on appropriate forums (such as alt.support.depression) generally receive rapid responses. Internet users have saved lives by counseling people online. Still, if you or a loved one is actively suicidal, look to a local suicide hotline or mental health professional for help—don't depend on the Internet or other online services.

Finally, keep in mind that no one is obligated to answer you. Healthcare professionals give online information, advice, and assistance because they want to. Don't take advantage of their altruism by demanding too much of their time. Don't flood them with e-mail or keep asking questions best directed to your own doctor. Physicians and other medical professionals who respond to posted queries usually do so with great care. The intent is usually to steer the individual in the right direction for additional offline medical assistance. No responsible healthcare professional wants you to use his or her online advice in place of that of your own doctor.

Finding the right group

You've checked the commercial services. You've searched the Web. You've logged onto BBSs. You can't find just the right group. Well, you still have a few options. If you use an Internet service provider that supports user home pages, you can create your own WWW page as a resource for whatever disease or disorder you're concerned about. Examples from this book include Web pages for polio, repetitive strain injury, and amputees. If you're interested in creating your own page, look to your Internet provider for instructions for how to do it (the cost varies). You can also subscribe to Delphi, where you can start your own custom forum (see chapter 3, *Commercial online services*).

You can also start your own Usenet newsgroup, but you must convince others to join you. The best bet is to go to the newsgroup most closely matching your interest and ask if other people share your need. Many groups are sensitive about splintering. Before you even consider starting a group, read news.groups for a while to learn how (and which) new groups are formed. To form a new newsgroup, there are requests for discussion and then a call for votes. Forming a new group is not an overnight process. Even if you initiate a new group, it won't necessarily be available everywhere on the Internet. That's up to system administrators all over the world.

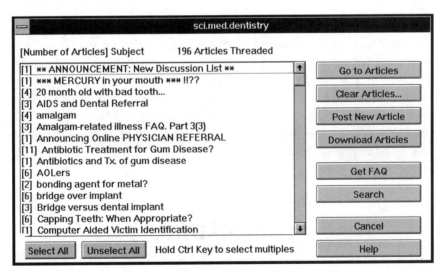

You'll often find new group announcements online.

Another option is to launch your own informal mailing list by announcing that you're starting a discussion group about disease X and want interested people to send you e-mail. Then you'll be responsible for collecting all messages, bundling them into a single digest, and mailing them back out to your subscribers. If the group really takes off, you can petition a site with Listserv or other automated software to carry your mailing list.

18
Special considerations

Going online for medical information is a new experience for most people. You'll probably find resources and treatments you've never heard of. You'll find scientific proof for some treatments and only anecdotal evidence for others. You need to take time to sift through the facts. In addition to evaluating the validity of online medical claims, you have to consider the impact of your own cyberspace communications. Sitting in front of a lifeless monitor and keyboard, you might not realize how many people can and will read whatever you write online. What you say could well influence others and have repercussions in your own life.

Clinical trials

On the Internet or commercial services, you might hear about clinical trials for new drugs or treatment protocols. If you're a patient looking for news of clinical trials, OncoLink provides information about new studies examining cancer treatments. Many disease-specific Web sites also alert visitors to researchers looking for patients. If you subscribe to CompuServe, the NORD database includes information about clinical trials for a number of diseases. Members of Usenet newsgroups and commercial service message boards also spread word about clinical trials. Simply because the clinical trial is advertised online, however, is no guarantee of its authenticity. And keep in mind that for some

Clinical Trials

- NCI Clinical Trials
- Novel Treatment of Brain Tumors - National Cancer Institute

- NCI's Clinical Trials Cooperative Group Program
- The National Cancer Institute Cancer Centers Program

OncoLink is just one site where you can find information about clinical trials.

patients, especially those with life-threatening diseases, these clinical trials—justifiably or not—raise hopes for improvement.

Some clinical trials examine new treatments, some test new drugs combined with old treatments, and some compare existing treatments. In addition, many clinical trials are blinded and randomized. That means if you participate in the clinical trial, there's no guarantee that you'll get the drug or treatment being tested. Instead, you might be part of a control group that gets no treatment (i.e., treatment with a placebo) or the old, standard treatment. In addition, many clinical trials are double blinded, which means even the researchers don't know who's in the test group and who's in the control group. This double blinding ensures that the researchers' or patients' preconceptions about one or another treatment won't affect the results of the study. If you don't want to risk being a control patient (with either no treatment or the old treatment), don't even call for information. You can't ask for the experimental treatment, so please don't try. Random selection decides who gets what treatment.

If you want to participate in a clinical trial, find out if it's a Phase I, II, or III trial. A Phase I trial determines the toxicity of the drug or treatment studied. A

Phase II trial determines the treatment's efficacy. In other words, does the drug or treatment work? A Phase III trial compares the treatment to standard therapies that already exist.

If you participate in a clinical trial and experience what you consider to be a strange side effect of the drug being tested, talk to the study researchers or coordinator. Since you won't know exactly what drug you're taking, going to the Internet for information is asking for trouble. In addition, the health professionals running the study need to be informed of every problem—no matter how trivial—that you experience. Your odd reaction to an experimental drug could be the 1 in 10,000 response that the researchers need to know about. If you look online for a solution instead of asking the clinical trial investigators, you might endanger your health and deprive the scientists of some important information. Be sure to also ask the study coordinator if you may discuss the study online before you post any messages.

Alternative treatments

Scientific methods can determine the safety and effectiveness of most medical treatments. Until recently, alternative medicine hasn't faced traditional scientific scrutiny, and claims for the effectiveness of alternative therapies have been based on anecdotal evidence. The arguments online for unproven treatments usually fall into the categories of "no scientific proof exists for its efficacy" and "true scientists can't just ignore this evidence." In the coming years, the Office of Alternative Medicine at the National Institutes of Health should begin to make headway in determining which alternative medical therapies really work. Until the results of the Office's research start coming in, no one can make absolute statements about the effectiveness (or ineffectiveness) of herbal treatments, macrobiotic diets, acupuncture, biofeedback, psychic healing, and so on.

In the meantime, let the buyer beware. Think carefully before you act on anecdotal evidence. The miraculous cure for your chronic problem might be snake oil. Of course, there's much information online about useful alternative healthcare, but the responsibility for researching claims is ultimately up to you.

If you're genuinely interested in an alternative treatment, take the time to investigate both online and offline. Ask focused questions in an appropriate discussion group. Some newsgroups are self-policing with regard to online treatment claims. A few dedicated members might do their own research and respond to any questionable postings by presenting as many facts as they can find. But don't count on getting "the rest of the story" online. If you want more information, correspond via e-mail with people whom you judge to be knowledgeable and reasonable. Question the credentials of anyone who makes a claim about a product or therapy. Ask that person to substantiate any claims with sources of additional information. Be an intelligent healthcare consumer.

What to expect from Net medicine

The difference between online medical advice and that which you get in your doctor's office is that you can't see whom you're speaking to online. The Internet is a broad church, and you'll find people ranging from those who believe that allopathic (modern) medicine is wrong and that only alternative medicine should be considered to those who believe the precise opposite.

The balance between alternative and allopathic advice depends to some extent on whether you ask your question in the alt. or in the sci. hierarchies. Once you've asked a question, you must wait to see what advice returns and then decide whom to believe. Sometimes you'll get no responses at all. This doesn't mean that your question is silly. It might simply be that it's very specialized and someone who knows about the topic hasn't seen it. It's therefore always worth reposting a question if there's no response after a week or so. If you get no response on the second attempt, it probably means no one is available who can help.

Sometimes you'll find that what you thought was a perfectly simple and innocent question will erupt into an almighty flame war, and your question will be lost in the static. When this happens, read the thread and decide whether you can believe any of the participants. Then e-mail them and explain that your question appeared to get lost in the fray but you still need help. Many of the medical participants on the Net will be happy to help in this situation.

You might find that you'll get useful advice from people who are being flamed heavily for their views. As a point of netiquette, they often appreciate a brief e-mail of support because many contributors get tired of constantly being attacked for giving out information. If they unsubscribe as a result, it's a great loss to all Net users because the range of available opinion is diminished. Just one letter of support makes contributing feel worthwhile.

Remember: Most of the professionals who give advice on the Net do it because they enjoy it!

Dr. Tim Reynolds
TimReyno@burton.demon.co.uk

Rights and responsibilities

Although the legal landscape of online medicine is far from clear, many laws regulating speech, print, and medicine can apply in cyberspace as well. The online community actively discourages smearing reputations of individuals of any stripe. Posted messages have an international audience, and you should be concerned about libel, defined as a false statement about someone that causes injury to his or her reputation. You'll hear discussion in some groups about unpleasant experiences with the medical profession. Be careful if you mention individuals by name. In fact, some discussion groups don't even permit mentioning another person's name—even in a positive context—without the permission of that person.

When taking information from another source, give credit to the creator of the original text or graphic. When posting excerpts or the full text of newspaper articles, journal articles, and other published material, list the full reference and clearly separate the quoted material from your own comments. This guideline also applies to information taken from a FAQ or other online document. Also, never post information publicly that was sent to you privately via e-mail unless you have the author's permission.

You can be held legally accountable for what you say online on message boards, newsgroups, and e-mail. Many online services archive all postings for their own protection. To protect themselves from legal liability, many medical professionals append disclaimers to their online communications. The disclaimer is for the author's protection, not yours. Before acting on information you receive online, independently verify it by asking your doctor, running a MEDLINE search, or checking other sources online and offline.

Finally, look to cyberspace as a resource, not as the last word. You can't depend on information or opinions you read online. Instead, integrate your online information with what you obtain from your doctor and from your own independent research. Don't relinquish control of your healthcare to individuals who haven't examined you, who don't know the full details of your medical history, and who won't be held accountable for what you do with their advice. In the end, the direction of your healthcare is up to you.

19
Sharing with your doctor

W hen you feel that you're ready to talk to your personal physician about what you've learned online, prepare for the exchange in several ways:

Decide which information is most important Don't flood your doctor with documents that, although interesting, might not help him or her evaluate the questions raised by your case. If you have a lot of information, bring only the most pertinent documents to your appointment. If you want to share messages from online bulletin boards, remember that postings from physicians probably will interest your doctor more than those from patients. If you really want to impress your doctor, bring medical literature citations and abstracts from a MEDLINE search. The last thing he or she wants is to know less than you.

Don't rely on your memory You don't want to omit any key facts. Giving your doctor printed material also gives him or her time to review the information outside the time pressures of a full clinic schedule.

Send the information in advance Depending upon your doctor's preference, send your research via U.S. mail, e-mail, or fax, along with a brief note explaining where you did your research and what questions you have. Your doctor will appreciate your consideration and might even read the material before you get there.

Request extra time with your doctor Don't try to cram a 30-minute discussion into a 10-minute office appointment.

Whatever you do, don't be afraid to share your online research with your doctor You're taking an active role in your treatment, and your doctor should respect and appreciate the effort.

If your doctor isn't open to talking about your online research, give him or her a chance Some physicians have little experience with patients who take charge of their own health. You might need to educate your doctor about the benefits of working with an informed patient. If your repeated efforts to collaborate with your doctor fail and if he or she refuses to communicate, look for another physician.

How to approach your doctor with information from the Internet

Doctors have as diverse a set of personalities, biases, opinions, and approaches to new information as anyone else, so there's really no sure-fire way to approach your own doctor. Some doctors get offended by questions and follow a "take it or leave it" approach with their patients. However, some doctors are very open to new information. I would recommend taking the following steps when you bring new Internet medical information to your doctor:

- Make sure your doctor has time to go over the information with you. If you're booked for a quick, post-operative visit, your doctor might be rushed and you won't get the full consideration you need. When booking the appointment, let the office clerk know that you have new information and questions that need answers.

- Be prepared. Read over the information ahead of time, and write down your specific questions. Organize the data you bring to highlight the specific issues you want to raise. Don't expect your doctor to be thrilled to wade through pages of unedited, repetitive threads.

- Take notes. You might want to feed your doctor's comments back into the Internet. Accuracy is important.

- Don't be surprised by a negative response. There's a lot of good information but also much misinformation on the Internet. You're equally likely to give your doctor valuable new information about your condition as you are to ask about the latest tonic from a cyber snake-oil salesman.

Daniel Shoskes, M.D.
Assistant Professor of Urology, UCLA

A
Internet reference books

*T*his book has focused entirely on online health and medical resources. You don't have to. If you'd like to explore the nooks and crannies of the Internet and become a power user, you might want to consider a reference book that reviews cyberspace in more detail. Always look for the most recent books, which will address the newest software and tools available—every day the Internet gets easier to use. You can start by flipping through these guides to see which one matches your level of understanding and method of Internet access:

Engst, Adam C. 1994. *Internet Starter Kit for Macintosh*, 2nd ed. Indianapolis, Ind.: Hayden Books.

Engst, Adam C., Corwin S. Low, and Michael A. Simon. 1995. *Internet Starter Kit for Windows*, 2nd ed. Indianapolis, Ind.: Hayden Books.

Kent, Peter. 1994. *The Complete Idiot's Next Step with the Internet*. Indianapolis, Ind.: Alpha Books.

Krol, Ed. 1994. *The Whole Internet User's Guide and Catalog*. Sebastopol, Calif.: O'Reilly & Associates.

Levine, John R. and Carol Baroudi. 1995. *Internet Secrets*. Foster City, Calif.: IDG Books.

Levine, John R. and Margaret Levine Young. 1994. *More Internet for Dummies*. Foster City, Calif.: IDG Books.

Smith, Richard J. and Mark Gibbs. 1994. *Navigating the Internet*. Indianapolis, Ind.: Sams Publishing.

B
Navigation tips

*I*n part 2 of this book we directed you to what we consider the most helpful sites for medical information. Out of hundreds of possible choices, we've selected listings that we consider not only the best, but also the most well-maintained. This means you'll be less likely to find outdated material, nearly empty directories, or menus "under construction." Before you start, though, you might want to read the following tips to keep from getting lost in the Internet's constantly changing landscape.

Many academic institutions and research facilities maintain gopher or Web servers mainly to help their employees get onto the Internet rather than let outside individuals in. The server of a well-known university or medical center might have disappointingly few resources. In addition, some features will be open only to individuals working at that particular institution.

When you arrive at a promising site for medical information, you might find only one or two documents in each directory. Often the usefulness and completeness of a particular resource depends on a single motivated individual who might move or lose enthusiasm or funding. Online resources are constantly evolving. If a particular site disappoints you, check again later and you might find a wealth of information and support.

Navigation tips

If you can't reach an address, don't give up. Try again an hour later or another day. The computer at that site might be having temporary problems or be disconnected from the Internet so the owners can do a backup or preventive maintenance. Other popular sites might be sluggish or inaccessible because so many people are using them at the same time.

If you can't get to a resource at the address we supply, see if a new address flashes up in the "can't access" message. Computer managers on the Internet often move files, sometimes entire computers. Many sites are now switching to Web service, which often changes their gopher address. If a site has moved, the owners will usually leave directions to help you find the new address. If not, consult chapter 15, *Searching for medical resources*, for tips for tracking down resources. You can also reach many resources, especially gopher servers, through alternative paths.

On the WWW, you might get a message that the URL entered doesn't exist. Before concluding you have the wrong address, try to access the site with a different Web browser. Netscape and Mosaic, both available at no charge on the WWW, can access almost every Web address.

If you have trouble connecting to the full address, don't use the information listed after the first single slash. For example, if the address http://www.cis.ohio-state.edu/hypertext/faq/usenet/powerlines-cancer-FAQ gives you trouble, just use http://www.cis.ohio-state.edu/ and then work your way through the appropriate directories to get the FAQ.

If you don't have WWW access and see an address that starts gopher://, leave off the gopher:// and use the rest of the address with your gopher software. You can try the same thing with addresses that start with http://. For most addresses, you can also usually identify the state or country in which the gopher server is located. You can then try to transfer to the gopher through the All the Gophers Servers in the World directory carried by the University of Minnesota and many other gopher servers.

If you're stuck, wait at least five minutes. Making both national and international connections can take a long time, especially during prime hours (roughly

7 A.M. to 7 P.M. Eastern time in the United States). In the evening, heavy consumer use and scheduled conferences jam many commercial services. If your gopher software, Web browser, commercial online software, or other connection software fails to make a connection, it will give up and tell you so. If you're stalled, try hanging up or turning off your modem, or even rebooting your computer. In any case, avoid trying to make the same failed connection right away.

All telephone numbers we list in this book are for modem use unless otherwise noted by the addition of (voice) after the number. Unless we give special instructions, use the standard communication protocol of 8-1-N.

To access all commercial service sites, you must pay at least a standard subscription charge. Because rates change constantly, we don't provide cost information (except for information retrieval services included in chapter 4, *Sample search for online medical information*). For resources available on the major commercial services, we add a ($) if the resource is part of an extended services option and ($$) if you pay extra charges on top of your regular subscription and online charges.

Abbreviations

Here are abbreviations of many of the computer terms and medical resources mentioned frequently in this book. We explain many of them in more detail in part one, *How to access online medical resources*.

ADA Americans with Disabilities Act (other organizations with the same acronym are written out)

BBS Bulletin board system (dial up with modem)

CDC Centers for Disease Control and Prevention

FAQ Frequently asked questions (a single document answering common questions)

FDA Food and Drug Administration

FTP File transfer protocol (for copying files from the Internet to personal computer)

HTML Hypertext mark-up language (used to add surfing links to documents)

HTTP Hypertext transport protocol (Web surfing protocol)

IRC Internet relay chat (real-time, live conversations with people around the world)

JAMA *The Journal of the American Medical Association*

NCI National Cancer Institute

NIAID National Institute of Allergies and Infectious Diseases

NIDDK National Institute of Diabetes and Digestive and Kidney Diseases

NIH National Institutes of Health

NORD National Organization for Rare Disorders

PDQ Physician Data Query (NCI's clinical trial database for physicians and patients)

QWK Software for downloading and reading mail and messages from BBSs

URL Universal resource locator (Internet address)

WHO World Health Organization

WWW World Wide Web (you can browse it with hypertext links)

C

Online resources for healthcare professionals

*P*hysicians and other healthcare professionals will find most of the resources described in part 2 of this book, *Where to find online medical resources*, useful. However, you might want to look at dozens of other sites that are more clinical or scientific in nature. You'll find multimedia textbooks, case studies, image libraries, databases, continuing education courses, employment services, and software centers geared toward healthcare professionals of all specialties. Several mailing lists open only to medical professionals are also available.

Be sure to check the central lists of online medical sites described in chapter 15, *Searching for medical resources*. In particular, Medical Matrix is designed for use by physicians and other professionals. New resources are announced in MMatrix (listserv@kumchttp.mc.ukans.edu), and MedWeb offers a comprehensive and well-organized index to biomedical Internet resources.

Finally, forums on the commercial services often have a discussion group or category that's limited to healthcare professionals; GEnie's Medical RoundTable has several medical professional categories that require application for admission. A few that are devoted entirely to medical personnel are listed later in this appendix.

We've suggested a few locations at the top of the list that you might want to use as starting points for your search for specialized information. If you're new to online resources and the use of computers in medical practice, be sure to look for Dr. Bruce McKenzie's Computers in Medicine file, which is posted regularly to sci.med. In general, the sci.med newsgroup is the best place to ask about online resources for medical professionals, and most new sites are announced here.

From our list, you'll want to visit Jim Martindale's Health Science Guide '95: A Health Science Multimedia Education and Specialized Information Resource Center. Here you'll find several virtual centers: medical, dental, veterinary, pharmacy, nursing, public health, nutrition, and allied health, plus access to The Reference Desk. Martindale's Virtual Medical Center includes a link to the LUMEN, another must-see. CHORUS, indexed by organ system and interconnected via hypertext links, serves as an online quick reference for information about diseases, radiological findings, and differential diagnoses for physicians and medical students. Physicians' Online is offered as a free medical information service (including free MEDLINE and other medical database searches) "by physicians for physicians." If you're looking for employment or someone to fill a medical-related position, be sure to check MedSearch America.

I've analyzed the Internet from the perspective of a busy family practitioner. There is a tremendous value in Internet networking and clinical information sharing with the Mosaic interface. There are also many hurdles to overcome. I've been involved with introducing the Internet to medical practitioners for some time and have accumulated a number of specific problems and solutions to the difficulty of getting clinicians on the Net:

Problem #1 Difficult interface

Solution #1 Introduce the Internet only when Mosaic-type browsers are available. All other uses are beyond the patience of busy practitioners.

Problem #2 Little useable content

Solution #2 HTML resource guides open up the resources. Specific resources that need support and maintenance include:

- Up-to-date treatment protocols (such as CancerNet)
- Practice guidelines (AHCPR)
- Employment databases
- Bulletin-boarding on practice issues, but moderation of the boards and operational guidelines need to be addressed.

Problem #3 Inadequate bandwidth

Solution #3 Telemedicine will be the richest framework for healthcare worker networking. Acceptance should parallel that of fax machines. Medical documents are nonstandard, nondigital, or formatted. High-bandwidth, encrypted interfacility transmissions could take place in 5 to 10 years.

Problem #4 Need better tools, more people online

Solution #4 Mosaic is adequate. Twenty dollars per month for unlimited access assures very rapid growth. Healthcare workers need to be informed of these revolutionary developments.

Many come into medical Internet without realizing it's a frontier. In the future, practitioners will be able to solve previously unsolvable clinical problems by using global expertise. However, the online medical world must be developed. It will take a good deal of effort on the part of medical societies and specialty groups to support peer review, moderation, and training.

Although many newsgroups and mailing lists are public and might prevent physicians and nurses from speaking freely and exchanging ideas, others are private. It's simple for the moderator to require biographical information. Medical practitioners are increasingly accepting of this.

It's useful to examine what has been accomplished in the psychiatry field with the InterPsych service. There are more than 20 professionally maintained mailing lists, a high-quality newsletter, an editorial board, an administration, etc.

Resources are developing rapidly. I'm the coauthor with Lee Hancock of a document called The Medical List, which presents clinical medicine resources as well as an HTML rendering of the same information (addresses following). I invite anyone seeking updated information about what medical resources are currently available on the Internet to check here first.

Gary Malet, D.O., Family Physician (gmalet@surfer.win.net)
The Medical List and Medical Matrix

Starting points

CHORUS (Collaborative Hypertext Resource): http://chorus.rad.mcw.edu/chorus.html
College of Medicine at the University of Florida: http://www.med.ufl.edu/
LUMEN (Loyola University Medical Education Network): http://www.meddean.luc.edu/lumen
Martindale's Health Science Guide '95 http://www-sci.lib.uci.edu/-HSG/HSGuide.html
Medical Resource Directory at UC Irvine: gopher://peg.cwis.uci.edu:7000/11/gopher.welcome/peg/MEDICINE
MedSearch America: http://www.medsearch.com/
Physicians' Online: 800-332-0009 (voice)
Primary care teaching topics: http://uhs.bsd.uchicago.edu/uhs/topics/uhs-teaching.html
SANTEC Web pages: http://www.santel.lu

Anesthesiology

Anest-L: listserv@ubvm.cc.buffalo.edu
GASNet (Global Anesthesiology Server Network): http://gasnet.med.nyu.edu/HomePage.html
University of Michigan Medical Center Department of Anesthesiology: http://www.anes.med.umich.edu/anes/

Bioethics

Bioethics Online Service: http://www.mcw.edu/bioethics or
gopher://post.its.mcw.edu:72/ or telnet://min.lib.mcw.edu or 414-266-5777
(At the prompt MCW, type C MIN, hit Enter, and choose the Bioethics Online
Service from the menu.)
Biomed-L: listserv@vm1.nodak.edu
bit.listserv.biomed-l

Dentistry

The Bridge: 415-368-2778
Dental_CE: listproc@bite.db.uth.tmc.edu
Dentalma: listserv@ucf1vm.cc.ucf.edu
Dentalweb: listproc@bite.db.uth.tmc.edu
Dentistry: dentisry@stat.com (Send e-mail to the list with your name and
address.)
Periodont: periodont@krypta.snafu.de (Type ADD in the subject line and
describe your involvement in the dental profession.)
WHOoral-Pilot (WHO Oral Health Group): mailbase@mailbase.ac.uk

Education

American Medical Student Association: gopher med-amsa.bu.edu or
http://med-www.bu.edu/AMSA
Erick's Guide to Medical School Admissions: http://homepage.seas.upenn.
edu/~santos/MedGuide.html
The Interactive Medical Student Lounge: http://falcon.cc.ukans.edu/~nsween
Medstu-L: listserv@unmvm.edu
Metronome Press (continuing medical education resources): gopher://
metronome.com/1
misc.education.medical
Misc.Education.Medical WWW Page: http://www.primenet.com/
~gwa/med.ed/memhome.html

Multimedia Medical Reference Library: http://www.tiac.net/users/jtward/index.html

Emergency medicine/trauma

Code-3 (Delphi): go CUSTOM 004
Emergency Services:http://dumbo.lsc.rit.edu/ems/index.html
Emergency Services WWW Site List: http://gilligan.uafadm.alaska.edu/www_911.htm
Global Emergency Medicine Archives : http://solaris.ckm.ucsf.edu:8081
TraumaNet (trauma and surgical critical care): http://www.trauma.lsumc.edu/

Environmental

Emflds-L: listserv@ubvm.cc.buffalo.edu
Occ-Env-Med-L: mailserv@mc.duke.edu

Epidemiology

Comprehensive Epidemiological Data (Lawrence Berkeley Laboratory): gopher://cedr.lbl.gov/

General practice

Family-L: listserv@mizzou1.missouri.edu
General Practice On Line: http://www.cityscape.co.uk/users/ad88/gp.htm
Health-L: listserv@irlearn.ucd.ie
Hippocrates: http://planetree1.utmem.edu/
Medical Forum (U.K. Delphi): go FORUM 18
UCSF's Division of General Internal Medicine: http://dgim-www.ucsf.edu/

Genetics

Baylor College of Medicine Genome Center: http://gc.bcm.tmc.edu:8088/
Baylor College of Medicine Tumor Gene Database: gopher://mbcr.bcm.
tmc.edu/oncogene.html
Hum-Molgen: listserv@nic.surfnet.nl
National Center for Biotechnology Information (GenBank): http://
www.ncbi.nlm.nih.gov/

Hematology/oncology

Bloodcell: majordomo@scripps.edu
Peter O'Connell Laboratory Breast Cancer Information Page:
http://mars.uthscsa.edu/POClab/Cancer/

Hospital administration

Healthmgmt: listserv@chimera.sph.umn.edu
Hspnet-L: listserv@uasc2.bitnet

Immunology

American Association of Immunologists: gopher://gopher.faseb.org:
70/11/Societies or http://www.aai.org or gopher://xerxes.nas.edu:
70/11/cwse/discipline/Immunology
sci.med.immunology
Tx-L (Transplant/Immunology Research List): listserv@anima.nums.nwu.edu

Medical informatics

American Medical Informatics Forum (CompuServe): go MEDSIG ($)
Artificial Intelligence & Medicine: ai-medicine-request@vuse.vanderbilt.edu

Artificial Intelligence in Medicine: ai-medicine-request@med.stanford.edu
Compumed: listserv@sjuvm.stjohns.edu
Health and Medical Informatic Digest: hmid-request@maddog.fammed.
wisc.edu
Medical informatics: http://galaxy.einet.net/galaxy/Medicine/Medical-
Technologies/Medical-Informatics.html
Medical informatics home pages: http://www-camis.stanford.edu/ or
http://dmi- www.mc.duke.edu/ or http://paella.med.yale.edu/
Medical informatics academic programs: http://www-
camis.stanford.edu/academics/informaticsprgms.html
Medinf-L: listserv@vm.gmd.de
Mednets: listserv@vm1.nodak.edu
MMatrix: listserv@kumchttp.mc.ukans.edu
The Piglet System (Personalized Intelligently Generated Explanatory Text,
online patient records): http://www.dcs.gla.ac.uk/~mercerlm/pigstart.html
sci.med.informatics
SMDM-L (Society for Medical Decision Making):
listserv@dartcms1.dartmouth.edu

Medical physicists

Health Physics Forum (Delphi): go CUSTOM 266
Medphys: medphys-request@radonc.duke.edu
Nucmed: nucmed-request@uwovax.uwo.ca
sci.med.physics

Minority health

Minhlth: minhlth-request@family.hampshire.edu

Neurology

Journal of Neurophysiology (contents only): gopher://oac.hsc.uth.
tmc.edu:3300/11/publications/jn/
Massachusetts General Hospital Department of Neurology: http://
132.183.145.103/
Neuro1-L: listserv@uicvm.uic.edu

Nursing

American Journal of Nursing Network: telenet ajn.org or 212-582-8137
Culture-and-Nursing: majordomo@itssrv1.ucsf.edu
Duke University Medical Center: http://nursing-
www.mc.duke.edu/nursing/nshomepg.htm
Gradnrse: listserv@kentvm.kent.edu
Nightingale Nursing Gopher: gopher://nightingale.con.utk.edu/
Nrsing-L: listproc@nic.umass.edu
NURSE WWW Information Service: http://www.csv.warwick.ac.uk:8000/
Nurse-UK: nurse-uk-request@warwick.ac.uk
Nursenet: listserv@vm.utcc.utoronto.ca
Nurseres: listserv@kentvm.kent.edu
Nursing Forum (U.K. Delphi): go FORUM 54
Nursing Network Forum (Delphi): go CUSTOM 261
Nursing Network Forum: nurse@access.digex.net
Nurse's Station (Delphi): go CUSTOM 046
Nursing Student's Recovery Room (Delphi): go CUSTOM 377
Ohio State University: http://www.con.ohio-state.edu/
Schlrn-L: listsrv@ubvm.cc.buffalo.edu
sci.med.nursing
Snurse-L: listserv@ubvm.cc.buffalo.edu
University of Washington School of Nursing:
http://www_son.hs.washington.edu/

Obstetrics/gynecology

Fet-Net: listserv@hearn.nic.surfnet.nl
Midwife: midwife-request@csv.warwick.ac.uk
Midwifery Internet Resources:
http://www.csv.warwick.ac.uk:8000/midwifery
OB-GYN-L: listserv@bcm.tmc.edu
Prenat-L: listserv@albnydh2.bitnet
Reprendo: listserv@umab.umd.edu

Ophthamology/optometry

EyeLine BBS: 404-303-1697
Eyemov-L: listserv@spcvxa.spc.edu
Oopraym (ophthamologists only): listserv@ubvms.cc.buffalo.edu

Osteopathic medicine

Michigan State University College of Osteopathic Medicine (MSUCOM)
Gopher Server: gopher://gopher.com.msu.edu:70/1/

Pathology

Pathology World Wide Web server: http://wwwpath.usuf2.usuhs.mil
sci.med.pathology
University Of Michigan Department of Pathology: http://zapruder.pds.
med.umich.edu/
University of Washington Department of Pathology: http://larry.pathology.
washington.edu/index.html or http://www.pathology.washington.edu/

Pharmacology/pharmacy

Formulary Exchange Service: 301-657-2617
Idaho State University College of Pharmacy: http://pharmacy.isu.edu/

MSB-L (Medical Sciences Bulletin Mailing List): msb-l-request@hslc.org
Pharm: pharm-request@DMU.AC.UK
Physician's GenRx International: http://www.icsi.net/GenRx or telnet
genrx.icsi.net [login: GENRX, password: GENRX]
PPS On-Line: http://www.pps.ca/pps.htm
Welsh School of Pharmacy: http://orchid.phrm.cf.ac.uk/
World List of Schools of Pharmacy: http://orchid.phrm.cf.ac.uk/WWW-
WSP/SoPListHomePage.html

Physician assistants

PA Page: http://www.halcyon.com/physasst/

Physiology

American Physiological Society: gopher://eja.anes.hscsyr.edu/
Thphysio (thermal physiology): listserv@frmop11.cnusc.fr

Psychiatry/psychology

Drugabus: listserv@umab.umd.edu
InterPsych (academic conferences):
http://www.psych.med.umich.edu/psychiatry/interpsych.html
InterPsych Thanatology Group: listserv@netcom.com
Neuro-Psych: listserv@netcom.com
Psyche (Interdisciplinary Journal of Research on Consciousness): http://
psyche.cs.monash.edu.au/
Psychological Resource List (academic): http://psych.hanover.edu/#contents
Psychopharmacology: listserv@netcom.com
Psychotherapy: listserv@netcom.com
Psycoloquy: listserv@pucc.princeton.edu
Psycoloquy home page:
http://www.w3.org/hypertext/DataSources/bySubject/Psychology/
Psycoloquy.html

Public health

Public-Health: mailbase@mailbase.ac.uk
Prevention Primer: http://www.health.org/primer/toc.html

Radiology

alt.images.medical
German Cancer Research Center (PET images): http://www.dkfz-heidelberg.
de/pet/home.htm
Milton S. Hershey Medical Center Department of Radiology: http://www.
xray.hmc.psu.edu/
Radsig: listserv@uwavm.u.washington.edu
Radsci-L: listserv@western.tec.wi.us
Radiological Society of North America: http://www.rsna.org/index.html
sci.med.radiology

Respiratory therapy

Respiratory Care World on Delphi: go CUSTOM 169

Risk assessment/insurance

RISKWeb: http://riskweb.bus.utexas.edu/riskweb.html

D
Medical FAQs (frequently asked questions)

As we've said throughout this book, you can probably find answers to many of your health-related questions in FAQs (frequently asked question files) prepared by medical discussion groups. You'll find these FAQs posted regularly in newsgroups or related Web pages or gopher servers.

We've listed here a sampling of the medical and health-related FAQs available online, including where to look for them. You can check a few central sources (we suggest four) for these existing FAQs as well as any new ones that have been developed recently. The misc.answers and news.answers newsgroups serve as the central Usenet posting locations for FAQs.

Medical FAQ List

ftp://ftp.demon.co.uk/pub/misc/MedFAQ.txt

Dr. Bruce McKenzie provides an invaluable service to the medical online community by maintaining the Medical FAQ List, which includes pointers to medical, health, and support-related FAQs on Usenet. You'll see the Medical FAQ List posted regularly to sci.med.

FAQ depository

ftp://rtfm.mit.edu/pub/usenet/news.answers/

In the FAQ depository you'll find official FAQs posted by medical newsgroups. These FAQs are also posted to appropriate Usenet newsgroups. The section later in this appendix, *Medical FAQs*, lists the directory paths for the FAQs at this site (MIT). For example, you would enter ftp://rtfm.mit.edu/pub/usenet/news.answers/abdominal-training to retrieve the Abdominal Training FAQ.

Hypertext FAQs

http://www.cis.ohio-state.edu/hypertext/faq/usenet/FAQ-List.html

At this Web site you'll find FAQs that have been converted from plain text to HTML. FAQs are listed alphabetically and can be searched by keyword.

misc.kids FAQ index

http://www.Internet-is.com/misc-kids/index.html

At this Web site you'll find the index to and hypertext versions of many of the health-related FAQs posted to misc.kids and misc.kids.health (check misc.kids. info as well). If you see any FAQs under *Medical FAQs* that are posted to misc. kids, try the misc.kids Web site too.

Medical FAQs

This section lists medical FAQs and their locations, by topic:

Abdominal training

misc.fitness
MIT: abdominal-training
http://www.dstc.edu.au/RDU/staff/nigel-ward/abfaq/abdominal-training.html

AIDS

sci.med.aids, sci.med
misc.health.aids, bionet.molbio.hiv
MIT: medicine/aids-faq
http://www.cis.ohio-state.edu/hypertext/faq/usenet/aids-faq/

Allergies/asthma

misc.kids

Alzheimer's disease

http://www.ncf.carleton.ca/go.html (select "alzheimer")

Amalgam

sci.med
http://www.algonet.se/~leif/AmFAQigr.html

Aneurysms

http://www.cc.columbia.edu:80/~mdt1/./

Arthritis

misc.health.arthritis

Asthma

sci.med, alt.med.allergy, alt.support.asthma
MIT: medicine/asthma/general-info

Asthma medications

sci.med, alt.support.asthma, alt.med.allergy
MIT: asthma/medications

Asthma resources

sci.med, alt.support.asthma

Attention deficit disorder (children)

misc.kids, alt.support.attn-deficit
http://www.seas.upenn.edu/~mengwong/add/add.fag.html

Autism

bit.listserv.autism
ftp://syr.edu/information/faqs/autism.faq

Bicycling

rec.bicycles.misc, ftp://draco.acs.uci.edu/rbfaq.html
MIT: bicycles-faq/
http://www.cis.ohio-state.edu/hypertext/faq/usenet/bicycles-faq/top.html

Birth planning

misc.kids.pregnancy
http://www.cis.ohio-state.edu/hypertext/faq/usenet/
misc-kids/pregnancy/birth-plan/top.html

Blood types/Rh incompatibility

misc.kids

Body building

misc.fitness
http://www.cis.ohio-state.edu/hypertext/faq/usenet/body-building/
hardgainer-faq/faq.html

Bradley method (childbirth, nutrition)

misc.kids.pregnancy
http://www.cis.ohio-state.edu/hypertext/faq/usenet/
misc-kids/preganncy/bradley/top.html

Brain injury

http://www.sasquatch.com/tbi

Caesarean section

misc.kids

Cancer

alt.support.cancer, sci.med.diseases.cancer
http://www.oncolink.upenn.edu/faq/
http://www.cis.ohio-state.edu/hypertext/faq/usenet/cancer-faq/faq.html

Chickenpox

misc.kids
http://www.cis.ohio-state.edu/hypertext/faq/usenet/misc-kids/chicken-pox/faq.html

Chronic fatigue syndrome (CFS)

alt.med.cfs, MIT: medicine/chronic-fatigue-syndrome/cfs-faq
Send GET CFS FAQ message to listserv%albnydh2@albany.edu

CFS electronic resources

alt.med.cfs
MIT: chronic-fatigue-syndrome/cfs-electronic-resources
Send GET CFS-NET TXT message to listserv@sjuvm.stjohns.edu

CFS (for medical professionals)

Send GET CFS-MED FAQ message to listserv@list.nih.gov

CFS network

alt.med.cfs, MIT:medicine/chronic-fatigue-syndrome/cfs-network-help
Send GET CFS NET-HELP message to listserv@sjuvm.stjohns.edu

CFS resources

alt.med.cfs, MIT: medicine/chronic-fatigue-syndrome/cfs-resources
Send GET CFS-RES TXT message to listserv@sjuvm.stjohns.edu

CFS treatments

alt.med.cfs, MIT: medicine/chronic-fatigue-syndrome/cfs-treatments
Send GET CFS-FAQ TREATMTS message to listserv%albnydh2@albany.edu

Circumcision (children)

misc.kids

Coffee and caffeine

http://daisy.uwaterloo.ca/~alopez-o/caffaq.html
http://www.cis.ohio-state.edu/hypertext/faq/usenet/caffeine-faq/faq.html

Colic (children)

misc.kids
http://www.cis.ohio-state.edu/hypretext/faq/usenet/misc-kids/colic/
faq.html

Collagenous colitis

alt.support.crohns-colitis
http://qurlyjoe.bu.edu/cducibs/colofaq.html

Cryonics

http://www.cs.cmu.edu
/afs/cs/user/tsf/Public-Mail/cryonics/html/overview.html
ftp://ftp.uu.net/usenet/news.answers/cryonics-faq
MIT: cryonics-faq/part*.Z

Depression

alt.support.depression
http://avocado.pc.helsinki.fi/~janne/asdfaq/

Depression book list

Self-Help Information Centre, SHIC@shic.com
alt.support.depression

Diabetes

misc.health.diabetes
http://www.cis.ohio-state.edu/hypertext/faq/usenet/diabetes/top.html

Diabetes (gestational)

misc.kids

Diabetes (juvenile)

misc.kids

Diabetes software

misc.health.diabetes

Diabetes (Type 2) oral medications

misc.health.diabetes

Diaper rash

misc.kids

Dieting

alt.support.diet
MIT: dieting-faq
Send SEND [ASD]ASD-FAQ*.TXT message to mailserv@vms.ocom.okstate.edu
http://www.cis.ohio-state.edu/hypertext/faq/usenet/FAQ-List.html

Dissociation

alt.support.dissociation
http://www.cis.ohio-state.edu/hypertext/faq/usenet/FAQ-List.html

Down's syndrome

http://fohnix.metronet.com/~thearc/faqs/down.html

Dystonia

alt.support.dystonia

Ear infections (children)

misc.kids

Eczema (children)

misc.kids
http://www.cis.ohio-state.edu/hypertext/faq/usenet/misc-kids/eczema/faq.html

Fat acceptance

alt.support.big-folks, soc.support.fat-acceptance
http://www.cis.ohio-state.edu/hypertext/faq/usenet/fat-acceptance-faq/top.html

Fibromyalgia

alt.med.fibromyalgia
Send GET FIBROM-L PT-FAQ mesage to listserv@vmd.cso.uiuc.edu
Send GET FIBROM-L MD-FAQ message to listserv@vmd.cso.uiuc.edu
Send GET FM-PAIN HANDOUT message to listserv@vmd.cso.uiuc.edu

Fitness

misc.fitness
http://www.cs.odu.edu/~ksw/mf-faq.html
http://www.cis.ohio-state.edu/hypertext/faq/usenet/misc-fitness/top.html

Homeopathic remedies

http://community.net/~neils/faqhom.html

Inflammatory bowel disease

alt.support.crohns-colitis
http://qurlyjoe.bu.edu/cducibs/ibdfaq.html
http://www.cis.ohio-state.edu/hypertext/faq/usenet/crohns-colitis-faq.html

Insulin pump

misc.health.diabetes

Irritable bowel syndrome

alt.support.crohns-colitis
http://qurlyjoe.bu.edu/cducibs/ibsfaq.html
MIT: medicine/irritable-bowel-syndrome-faq

Medical education

misc.education.medical, sci.med

Medical (general)

sci.med
ftp://ftp.demon.co.uk/pub/misc/MedFAQ.txt

Medical image formats

alt.image.medical
http://www.rahul.net/dclunie/medical-image-faq/html/
http://www.cis.ohio-state.edu/hypertext/faq/usenet/medical-image-faq/top.html

Medical informatics

sci.med.informatics
http://www.cis.ohio-state.edu/hypertext/faq/usenet/medical-informatics-faq/faq.html

Meditation

alt.meditation
http://www.cis.ohio-state.edu/hypertext/faq/usenet/meditation-faq/faq.html

Migraine

alt.support.headaches.migraine
http://www.cis.ohio-state.edu/hypertext/faq/usenet/alt.support.headaches.migraine/part1/faq.html

Medical FAQs (frequently asked questions)

Miscarriage

misc.kids
http://scalos.mc.duke.edu/~brook006/
http://www.cis.ohio-state.edu/hypertext/faq/usenet/misc-
kids/miscarriage/top.html

Multiple sclerosis

alt.support.mult-sclerosis
http://www.infosci.org/MS-Internat/Internat

Nursing

sci.med.nursing
http://www.csv.warwick.ac.uk:8000/sci.med.nursing.html

Oriental medicine

ftp://ftp.cts.com/pub/nkraft/ormed.html

Panic disorder

alt.support.anxiety-panic

Pediatrician (how to select one)

misc.kids
http://www.cis.ohio-state.edu/hypertext/faq/usenet/misc-kids/pediatrician-
questions/faq.html
Send message SEND PED FAQ to lchirlia@cc.brynmawr.edu

Personality types

http://sunsite.unc.edu/personality/

Power lines and cancer

sci.med.physics
ftp://cdmas.crc.mcw.edu/pub/Powerlines_and_cancer/
MIT: powerlines-cancer-FAQ/http://www.cis.ohio-state.edu/
hypertext/faq/usenet/powerlines-cancer-FAQ/top.html

Pregnancy (several topics)

misc.kids
http://www.cis.ohio-state.edu/hypertext/faq/usenet/misc-kids/pregnancy/top.html

Prenatal testing

misc.kids.info
MIT: misc-kids/pregnancy/screening/
http://www.cis.ohio-state.edu/hypertext/faq/usenet/misc-kids/pregnancy/sreening/top.html

Preterm birth

misc.kids

Prostatitis

alt.support.prostate.prostatitis

Psychology

sci.psychology
http://www.cis.ohio-state.edu/hypertext/faq/usenet/psychology-faq/faq.html

Psychology and support groups

sci.med

Recovery (addiction)

alt.recovery
ftp://ftp.netcom.com/pub/dh/dhawk/Recovery.html
http://www.moscow.com/Resources/SelfHelp/AA/
http://www.cis.ohio-state.edu/hypertext/faq/usenet/alt-recovery/welcome/faq.html

Recovery (alcoholism)

alt.recovery.aa
ftp://ftp.netcom.com/pub/dh/dhawk/AA.FAQ.html

http://www.cis.ohio-state.edu/hypertext/faq/usenet/alt-recovery/alcolholics-anonymous-faq/faq.html

Running

rec.running
MIT: running-faq/

Sexual abuse

alt.sexual.abuse.recovery

Sleep disorders

alt.support.sleep-disorders
http://www.access.digexnet/~faust/sidord/osa.faq.html

Smoking cessation

alt.support.stop-smoking
http://www.ncl.ac.uk/~nnpb/
http://www.swen.waterloo.ca/~bpekilis/AAS/Faq/a.s.s.-s_faq.html

Spina bifida

alt.support.spina-bifida

Static electromagnetic fields and cancer

http://www.cis.ohio-state.edu/hypertext/faq/usenet/
static-fields-cancer-FAQ/top.html

Stop smoking/clean air

alt.support.non-smokers.moderated

Stretching

misc.fitness
http://www.cis.ohio-state.edu/hypertext/faq/usenet/stretching/top.html

Stuttering

alt.support.stuttering
gopher://gopher.mankato.msus.edu/ (go to Academic Colleges &
Departments, then to Communication Disorders)

Sudden infant death syndrome

misc.kids
MIT: misc-kids/sids
http://www.cis.ohio-state.edu/hypertext/faq/usenet/misc-kids/sids

Suicide

alt.suicide.holiday
http://www.cis.ohio-state.edu/hypertext/faq/usenet/suicide/top.html

Surgery (children)

misc.kids

Surgery (myopia)

sci.med

Tinnitus

sci.med
ftp://ftp.cccd.edu/pub/faq/tinnitus.txt
http://www.ccd.edu/faq/tinnitus.html

Tourette's syndrome

alt.support.tourette

Training nutrition

sci.med.nutrition, misc.fitness
http://www.dgsys.com/~trnutr/FAQ

Transcendental meditation

alt.meditation.transcendental, sci.med

Transplantation

sci.med, bit.listserv.transplant
MIT: bit.listserv.transplant

Typing injury

sci.med
http://www.cs.princeton.edu/~dwallach/tifaq/
http://www.cis.ohio-state.edu/hypertext/faq/usenet/
typing-injury-faq/top.html

Vaccination (children)

misc.kids
http://www.cis.ohio-state.edu/hypertext/faq/usenet/
misc-kids/vaccinations/top.html

Vasectomy

sci.med

Vegetarianism

rec.foods.veg
http://catless.ncl.ac.uk/Vegetarian/
MIT: vegetarian/faq
http://www.cis.ohio-state.edu/hypertext/faq/usenet/vegetarian/top.html

Vision and eye care

sci.med; sci.med.vision
http://ucaussie.berkeley.edu/UCBSO.html
MIT: sci/
http://www.cis.ohio-state.edu/hypertext/faq/usenet/vision-faq/top.html

Index

Index

Index

Index

Index

Index

Index

About the authors

Educated at Yale (B.A.) and the University of California, San Francisco School of Medicine (M.D.), Dr. Tom Linden has been interested in communications since he could talk. He was an editor of the *Yale Daily News*, a staff writer for the *Los Angeles Times*, anchor of a weekly national medical news program on Lifetime Medical Television, and most recently medical editor for "Fox 11 News" and talk radio host for "710 Talk KMPC," both in Los Angeles. He's chairman of MedWorld Productions, Inc. and lives in Southern California with his family.

Freelance medical writer Michelle L. Kienholz has written for The American Dietetic Association, The NutraSweet Company, The International Life Sciences Institute, and many other organizations and publications. She has also worked as medical editor for the Nutrition/Metabolism Laboratory at Harvard Medical School's Deaconess Hospital, both in Boston and remotely from rural Virginia.

Your first stop on the Information Highway should be a place you can call home.

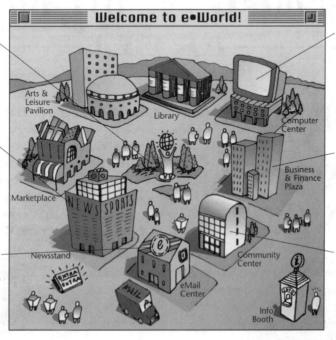

You already know how to get around.
Apple's simple graphic interface makes it easy to find information and navigate around eWorld.

All the news you want on your virtual doorstep.
eWorld offers up-to-the-minute news (even the latest sports scores) from wire services, newspapers and magazines from around the world.

The postman works all day, every day.
It's a snap to send electronic mail to users of eWorld and other electronic services, including the Internet.

Macintosh® support in your own backyard.
eWorld is your direct connection to support information from Apple and other software and hardware companies.

The experts live next door.
Business, financial and management insights are at your fingertips.

You'll want to meet your neighbors.
eWorld is a global community of thoughtful, respectful and inquisitive people who want to hear from you!

Check out your new neighborhood. Send for your eWorld for Macintosh Starter Kit and try ten hours free.

If you think navigating the Information Highway has to be confusing, you haven't spent time on eWorld,™ the on-line service from Apple.

eWorld is a totally different kind of on-line service. You feel at home right away, because eWorld was designed from the start to be easy to use. Information is organized intelligently, graphically and simply, so you can get to what you want quickly—without being overwhelmed. You also have access to great on-line support from Apple and other software and hardware companies. And the eWorld community is downright neighborly, with respectful, relevant and thoughtful on-line conversation.

eWorld is bustling with information for everyone's tastes: from educational activities for kids to tips for graphic designers to the latest from Hollywood and the sports world. But instead of telling you, we think you'd prefer to see for yourself. So send for your free eWorld Starter Kit, including software and special registration information—everything you need to sign on right away.

eWorld™
Apple's on-line service.

Ten FREE hours

To receive your free Starter Kit plus 10 hours free on-line, call 1 800 521-1515 ext. 410 or mail us this coupon.

Name _____

Company Name _____

Home Address _____ Apt./Suite # _____

City _____

State _____ ZIP _____

Phone ( ) _____

Check one: ☐ 1.4MB Disk ☐ 800K Disk

☐ Check here if you'd like to receive information about eWorld for Windows as it becomes available.

Return this coupon to:
eWorld Starter Kit
Apple Computer, Inc.
P.O. Box 4493
Bridgeton, MO 63044-9718

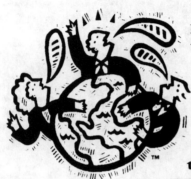

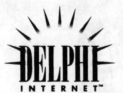

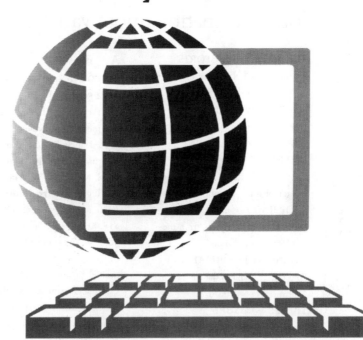

CompuServe
delivers more of what you want in an online service.

More information, more variety, more

NEWS/WEATHER/SPORTS
Keep informed of current events and the people who shape them.

ELECTRONIC MAIL
Stay in touch with friends, family, and associates around the world.

REFERENCE LIBRARIES
Uncover the facts you need in minutes, for personal use, school, or business.

SHOPPING
Shop, without dropping, from the comfort of your home.

FINANCIAL INFORMATION
Find timely financial data and realize your money's worth.

TRAVEL & LEISURE
Book trips with the same service used by professional travel agents.

ENTERTAINMENT
Enjoy a host of games, reviews, and newspaper columns.

INTERNET
Gain full access to The Internet ... including the World Wide Web.

Act now to receive a FREE introductory membership and software.

You'll get a free Membership Kit that includes everything you need to get started, including the CompuServe Information Manager software for DOS, Macintosh, or Windows. Plus, you'll **get one free month of our basic services** (worth $9.95), a $15.00 usage credit to explore our other services, and a free subscription to *CompuServe Magazine*. This is a limited-time offer available to new CompuServe members only. One special membership per person. Communication surcharges may apply in some areas.

To get connected to the world's most comprehensive online information service, call **1 800 524-3388** and ask for Representative 449. Outside the U.S. and Canada, call 614 529-1349.

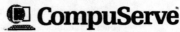

The information service you won't outgrow.